A Simple Guide to Orthopaedics

Dedication

To medical students — past, present and future.

A Simple Guide to Orthopaedics

R. L. Huckstep CMG, FTS, Hon MD (NSW)
MA MD(Cantab) FRCS(Edin) FRCS(Eng) FRACS FAOrthA

Professor and Head, Hugh Smith Department of Traumatic and Orthopaedic Surgery University of New South Wales and Emeritus Consultant, Orthopaedic Surgeon, Prince of Wales Hospital, Sydney, Australia; *Lately* Chairman of Orthopaedic Surgery and Director of Accident Services, Prince of Wales and Prince Henry Hospitals, Chairman or Member, various Accident and Disaster Committees in Australia and Senior Medical Disaster Commander, Sydney; *Lately* Chairman, School of Surgery, University of New South Wales, Vice-President, Australian Orthopaedic Association; Professor of Orthopaedic Surgery, Makerere University, Kampala, Uganda; Hunterian Professor, Royal College of Surgeons of England; Corresponding Editor, Journal of Bone and Joint Surgery, Injury and the Archives of Orthopaedic and Traumatic Surgery.

Editing, Formatting and Illustrations

M. D. Gardiner MB BS Hons. (NSW)

J. D. Greenstein BSc MB BS (NSW)

S. Hutabarat BSc MB BS (NSW)

G. Long MB BS (NSW)

J. S. Magnussen JP MB BS (NSW)

M. L. Miller

F. Rubiu

T. Tran MB BS (NSW)

CHURCHILL LIVINGSTONE

EDINBURGH LONDON MADRID MELBOURNE NEW YORK and TOKYO 1993

CHURCHILL LIVINGSTONE
Medical Division of Longman Group UK Limited

Distributed in the United States of America by Churchill Livingstone Inc., 650 Avenue of the Americas, New
York, N.Y. 10011, and by associated companies, branches
and representatives throughout the world.

FIRST PUBLISHED 1993

ISBN 0-443-04385-X

British Library of Cataloguing in Publication Data
A catalogue record for this book is available from the
British Library

Library of Congress Cataloging in Publication Data
A catalog record for this book is available from the
Library of Congress.

The
publisher's
policy is to use
paper manufactured
from sustainable forests

Produced by Longman Singapore Publishers (Pte) Ltd.
Printed in Singapore.

Preface

Many excellent books on orthopaedic surgery have been written for both the undergraduate and post-graduate. Most are too large and too detailed for busy undergraduates, junior doctors or general practitioners.

The general format of 'A Simple Guide to Orthopaedics' follows the author's book 'A Simple Guide to Trauma' which is now in its 5th edition and aims to provide a simply illustrated book which is comprehensive enough to cover the most common orthopaedic conditions.

This book has been written mainly for senior medical students, junior doctors working in outpatient and casualty departments and for general practitioners. It should also be of value to nurses and physiotherapists treating patients with orthopaedic problems.

Almost every page of text has a full facing page of simple illustrations, relevant to the text. The book has been divided into two sections. *Section I* is devoted to history, examination, investigation and treatment. *Section II* discusses specific orthopaedic conditions. In the first section, following the examination of each joint, examples are given of conditions which may affect that joint, with reference to the relevant chapters in Section II. A standard classification of orthopaedic conditions has been used throughout the book, namely: congenital abnormalities, neoplasia, trauma, infection, arthritis and paralysis.

Patient examination has been simplified to follow the excellent teaching of Mr A. G. Apley, and his format of Look, Feel and Move.

Section I is almost self-contained, and would be useful for the medical student beginning orthopaedics, as well as for nurses, physiotherapists and others as a simple illustrated guide to orthopaedic examination, investigation and treatment.

Section II expands on the first section and is designed for the more advanced student, the junior doctor and the general practitioner, while still being of value as a reference text for more senior staff. It has chapters on congenital and paediatric conditions, musculoskeletal neoplasms, infection, arthritis, neurological and spinal conditions, metabolic and endocrine bone disease, upper and lower limb conditions, and finally a summary of common orthopaedic conditions encountered in the elderly patient. Each of these chapters also includes an individual classification table for ease of reference.

Although traumatic conditions have been referred to, a specific chapter has not been included as this is covered in the author's companion volume 'A Simple Guide to Trauma'.

An appendix giving the reference intervals for common investigations in haematology and clinical chemistry has been included. This is followed by a list of references which includes other books recommended for the reader wishing to obtain further information.

The systematic division of the book has necessitated occasional repetition of information, but this is felt to be important in order to make each chapter relatively self contained. The index is comprehensive, for ease of reference, with the important page references in bold print and illustrations shown in italics, thus making a glossary of orthopaedic terms largely unnecessary.

Obviously a book of this size cannot cover all orthopaedic conditions, but despite this the most common, relevant and important topics have been included.

Acknowledgements

I am grateful to the various doctors, medical students and others who have helped in the publication of this book which has been written for them. Their advice on its format and content has always been carefully considered.

The formatting and editing of this book by Matthew Gardiner, John Magnussen and Michelle Miller has simplified its publication.

Several artists have been responsible for the simple, but clear illustrations. I would like particularly to acknowledge Jim Greenstein, Simon Hutabarat, Gareth Long, Franca Rubiu, Tuan Tran and Michelle Van Capelle.

I should also like to thank Mr Michael Oakey and his staff at the Medical Illustration Department, the Prince of Wales Hospital, Sydney, as well as the many students and staff who have contributed to the book and particularly: Peter Boers, Sue Connor, Bruce Cooper, Louise Delaney, Robin Diebold, Ali Gursel, Graeme Hall, Renee Hannan, Kate Harrison, Sally Hill, Michelle Hogg, Michael Huckstep, Bernard I'Ons, Mark Jackson, Michael Maley, Carl O'Kane, Mark Slockee, Ellie Tapp, Steve Thackway, Robert Turner and Olive Yanelli for their assistance.

I am also indebted to the late Dr Hugh Smith whose considerable assistance enabled my research department at the University of New South Wales to be founded.

Finally, as with my other books and publications over the past 30 years, I would like to thank my wife Ann for her patience and help. The staff of Churchill Livingstone and particularly Miss Clare Wood-Allum have been, as usual, most helpful in the publication of this book.

Sydney, 1992   R. L. Huckstep

A Simple Guide to Orthopaedics

Contents

Section I

Section II

A Simple Guide to Orthopaedics

Section I

History, Examination, Investigations, and Treatment

Chapter 1

History and Examination

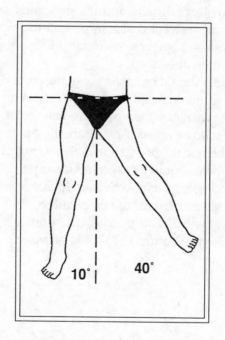

10°   40°

Orthopaedic History

An adequate history is essential before the patient is examined. This will give a clue to the diagnosis. It will also ensure that the most relevant part of the patient is examined. It may be categorised as is shown on the opposite page.

History of present illness

The present history should include questions about any pain, swelling, deformity, limitation of movement and also if these restrict normal activities.

The type of pain may be relevant, as well as its radiation proximally or distally, and any associated sensory or motor disturbances. It is also important to ask whether pain is increased by exercise and if it keeps the patient awake or interrupts sleep.

Questions should be asked about the parts distal and proximal to the affected area. Any extension of pain, numbness, weakness, temperature change or swelling distally should be noted. Any disabilities, pain or swelling elsewhere in the body should also be noted.

The patient should be asked about any treatment for a current complaint, its effectiveness, possible side effects, and an assessment made of compliance.

Finally, general and specific questions about other systems likely to be affected should be asked.

General Medical History

Identifying data: name, age, address, occupation

Presenting symptom(s)

History of present illness

Current treatment: effectiveness, side effects and compliance

Past medical and surgical history

Family history

Social and occupational history

Systems review

Past history

This should include questions regarding previous operations, illnesses or injuries, and also general health.

Family history

Details of the immediate family's health is an important part of the history. This should include medical and surgical illnesses in the patient's parents, siblings and children.

Social and occupational history

A social history should make brief reference to domestic, interpersonal, legal and financial matters. An occupational history is important since it has a bearing on the likely risk factors, approach to treatment and patient compliance.

A history of alcohol and other drug consumption is an essential part of the social history. An alcoholic, overweight, heavy smoker is much more likely to develop conditions such as lung carcinoma and hepatic cirrhosis. This patient is also more likely to have postoperative complications from surgery.

The way in which the patient gives a history, and even the past history, can provide a good indication as to whether the symptoms described are genuine, and the likelihood of patient response to treatment. The type of treatment given and the availability of domiciliary care may alter the necessity for hospitalisation.

Obtaining a history from a young child may be difficult. Parents may provide some information, and more reliance will need to be placed on physical examination.

A patient's occupation and ability to work may be relevant. A patient complaining of back pain, for instance may relate this to lifting heavy weights at work. This may

Systems Review

Cardiovascular system

Chest pain, dyspnoea, swollen ankles

Respiratory system

Cough, sputum, dyspnoea, fever

Central nervous system

Headaches, weakness, altered consciousness

Gastrointestinal system

Nausea, vomiting, abdominal pain, altered bowel habits

Genitourinary system

Frequency, dysuria, discharge, haematuria

Musculoskeletal system

Pain, restricted movement, past trauma

General

Weight loss, weakness, mental state

in turn be exaggerated, with a view to compensation payments or extended time off duty.

The type of work carried out by the patient may also be relevant to possible treatment. For example the management of back pain in someone in a sedentary occupation, who takes little exercise, may be viewed differently from that of someone whose job involves heavy lifting.

Aetiology of Orthopaedic Conditions

Congenital
1. Genetic eg. achondroplasia
2. Infection eg. rubella
3. Drugs eg. thalidomide
4. Radiation eg. X-rays
5. Trauma

Acquired
1. Neoplasia —
   benign
   malignant
2. Trauma —
   soft tissue
   fracture and dislocation
3. Infection —
   acute
   chronic
4. Arthritis —
   degenerative
   autoimmune
   metabolic
5. Paralysis —
   cerebral
   spinal
   peripheral
6. Miscellaneous — Paget's disease

Orthopaedic Examination

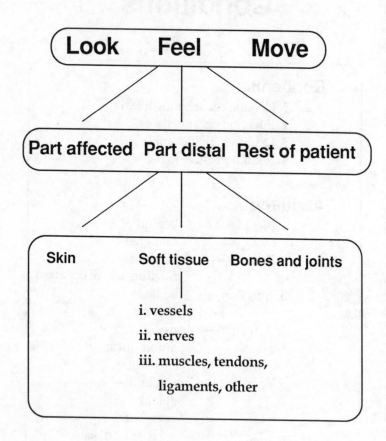

Look   Feel   Move

Part affected Part distal Rest of patient

Skin   Soft tissue   Bones and joints

i. vessels

ii. nerves

iii. muscles, tendons,

    ligaments, other

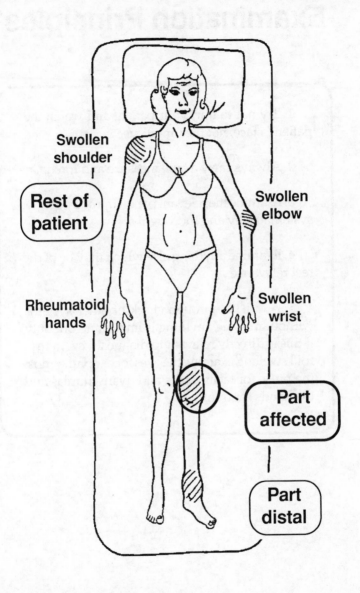

Swollen shoulder

Rest of patient

Swollen elbow

Rheumatoid hands

Swollen wrist

Part affected

Part distal

Examination Principles

1. Try not to hurt your patient and watch the patient's face, not the umbilicus.

2. Always carry a tape measure and torch.

3. Examine the relevant part of the body gently, systematically and thoroughly.

4. Examine anything else which may be of direct relevance.

5. A quick, thorough check of other systems without missing anything is important, but only if this is directly relevant to diagnosis, eg. in thyroid swelling examine the eyes for exophthalmos, the pulse for tachycardia and dysrhythmias and the hands for tremor.

The Part Affected

Look

1. Skin
2. Soft tissues — vessels
    nerves
    other eg. muscles, tendons,
    ligaments, fat, fascia, lymph nodes
3. Bone and joint including synovia and ligaments

Feel

Skin

The skin should be felt for — tenderness
    temperature
    fluctuation
    sensory disturbance

    It is important to compare both sides of the body, and to feel the front, back, and sides of the part affected.

Soft tissue

Soft tissue should be carefully palpated and abnormalities noted. Soft tissue examination can be divided into three sections:

    Vessels
    Nerves
    Other — muscle, tendons, ligaments
        fat, fascia, lymph nodes

Vessels

Abnormal or absent pulsation should be noted. An aneurysm can usually be moved from side to side rather than longitudinally, it may pulsate, and a bruit may be heard on auscultation. Examination of the distal part of

Look

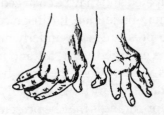

Rheumatoid hands

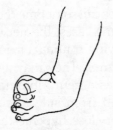

Talipes varus deformity

Feel

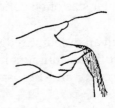

Axillary lymph nodes

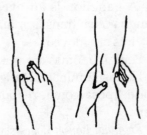

Patella and joint margins

Move

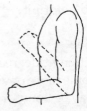

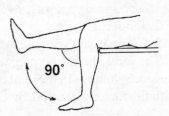

90°

the limb may highlight differences in appearance and temperature.

Nerves

Nerves can sometimes be palpated and may be enlarged. In some cases, the nerves may be tender, for instance following trauma, or due to pressure from underlying structures. They may also be enlarged with a tumour such as a neurofibroma. As with vessels, they can be moved from side to side rather than longitudinally. Sensory loss, hyperaesthesia or paralysis may be present in the distal part of the limb in nerve injuries.

Other structures

Muscles and tendons should be palpated for tenderness. Tendons may be shortened or ruptured.

A ganglion is an overgrowth of synovial tissue. Ganglia often transilluminate and their size often varies as joints are moved.

Benign lipomas are very soft with an indefinite edge and transilluminate. Malignant soft tissue tumours include liposarcoma, rhabdomyosarcoma and fibrosarcoma.

Regional lymph nodes should always be palpated for enlargement in all cases where there is a possibility of infection or neoplastic disease.

Bones and joints

These should be carefully palpated for:

1. Abnormal anatomy, swelling and deformity
2. Tenderness
3. Comparison with the opposite side

The joint should be palpated in different degrees of flexion. Swellings in the joint may become more obvious with flexion or extension. Swellings may be bony, or soft tissue, or both. If the swelling is soft tissue, it should be assessed as to whether it is:

1. Synovial tissue
2. Fluid —   synovial fluid
             blood
             pus
3. Both

Move

As well as testing the muscles, ligaments should be assessed where possible. This is particularly important in the knee and the ankle, where ligament laxity compromises weight-bearing.

Detailed examination of joints is discussed in subsequent pages. In children or apprehensive adults, active movements should be carried out before passive. Passive movements (movements gently carried out by the examiner) should always be assessed in addition to active movements (carried out by the patient).

Individual joints have different types of movement. Most joint movements, however, can be divided into three major components:

1. Flexion/extension
2. Abduction/adduction
3. Internal/external rotation

After assessing active and passive movements, the power of relevant muscle groups should be assessed.

The Part Distal

Look

The limb should be inspected for scars, deformities and also for any obvious shortening. It is important to examine the sides, back and front of the limb, and also to compare the opposite limb. Small differences in colour, swelling, wasting and deformity can only be noticed by careful comparison of the two sides.

Feel

A systematic examination of the limb affected will mean that nothing important is missed. The skin is felt for warmth. Any difference in sensation is compared with the opposite side and tender areas noted. The arterial pulses are palpated and compared, when appropriate, with the opposite side.

Move

The joint should be moved through its full range of movements:

1. Active movement — movement by the patient. In children, apprehensive patients, or in cases of suspected spinal injury, always carry out active movement before passive.
2. Passive movement — movement by the examiner
3. Power
4. Ligamentous stability

Look

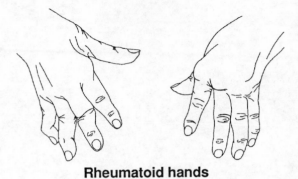

Rheumatoid hands

Feel

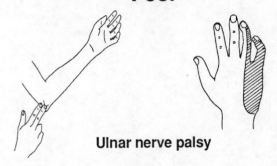

Ulnar nerve palsy

Move

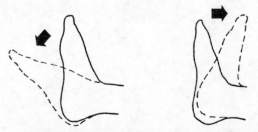

Ankle plantarflexion and dorsiflexion

A Simple Guide to Orthopaedics

The Rest of the Patient

Look

> 1. Opposite side
> 2. Head and neck
> 3. Trunk, spine and abdomen
> 4. Other limbs

Feel

> 1. Temperature
> 2. Tenderness
> 3. Abnormal masses

Move

> 1. Active
> 2. Passive
> 3. Ligamentous stability

Overall Examination

Head and neck

General inspection
Swellings, wasting, deformity, skin

Eyes
Pupils, conjunctivae, fundi

Ear, nose and throat

Neck
JVP, carotids, thyroid , lymph nodes, trachea

Upper limb

General inspection
Swelling, wasting, deformity

Pulse and blood pressure

Neurological examination
Tone, power, reflexes, sensation, co-ordination

Bone and joint examination

Precordium

General inspection
Swelling, wasting, deformity

Heart
Size, heart sounds, murmurs

Lungs
Breath sounds, additional sounds

Rib cage and breasts

Overall Examination

Back

General inspection
Swelling, wasting , deformity

Lungs

Spine
Scoliosis, kyphosis, tenderness

Movements

Abdomen

General inspection

Palpation
Liver, spleen, kidneys, other masses

Percussion and auscultation

Perineum
Herniae, lymph nodes (inguinal and femoral),
rectal and genital examination (if relevant)

Lower limb

General inspection
Swelling, wasting, deformity

Neurological examination
Tone, power, reflexes, sensation, co-ordination

Vascular examination
Pulses, temperature, ulceration, trophic changes

Bone and joint examination

Shortening and gait disturbance

Chapter 2

Examination of the Upper Limb

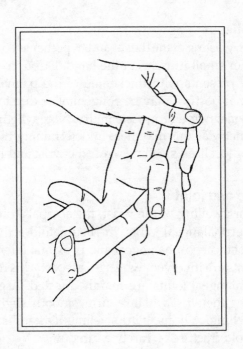

Hand and Wrist Examination

Look

1. General inspection
Look for any signs of asymmetry, abnormal posture, deformity or wasting.

2. Skin
Look for scars, sinuses or colour changes. Observe the nails for clubbing, pitting or other deformity.

3. Soft tissue
Look for wasting of the thenar and hypothenar eminences and other small muscles of the hand. Dupuytren's contracture presents with thickening of the palmar fascia. Abnormal posture may be congenital or due to a traumatic bone, nerve or muscle injury. Note whether there is symmetry as this may help in determining the cause. Look for localised swellings over the wrist and hand.

4. Bone and joint
Look for swelling of the wrist, metacarpals, phalanges and interphalangeal joints. In rheumatoid arthritis the wrist, metacarpo-phalangeal and proximal interphalangeal joints are involved, whilst in osteoarthritis the distal interphalangeal joints are mainly affected. A ganglion overlying the wrist will be a firm, smooth, slightly mobile swelling. A bony, hard swelling may indicate a recent or old fracture or, rarely, a tumour.

Hand and Wrist Examination

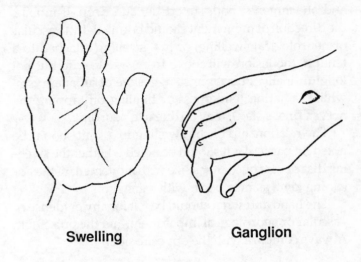

Swelling

Ganglion

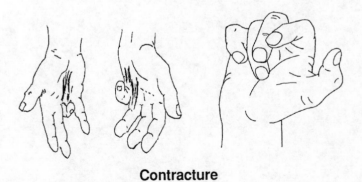

Contracture

Feel

The joint should be carefully palpated for any tenderness.

Swellings should be palpated for consistency, contour and attachments, both superficial and deep. If mobile, the direction of movement should be noted. In a vascular or neurological swelling, or in a swelling attached to a tendon, the lesion will move from side to side but not longitudinally. Pulsation is suggestive of an aneurysm, whilst radiating tenderness or tingling on tapping the nerve (Tinel's sign), may be due to a neuroma.

The relationship of the swelling to a joint should be noted. In particular it should be noted whether the swelling disappears or changes size with movement of the adjoining joint, as may occur with a ganglion.

The hand and wrist should be felt for any evidence of vascular or neurological impairment, and the pulses felt. Always compare with the opposite side.

Hand and Wrist Examination

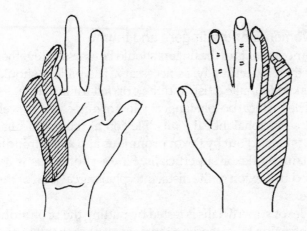

**Ulnar nerve palsy,
clawing, sensory loss, wasting**

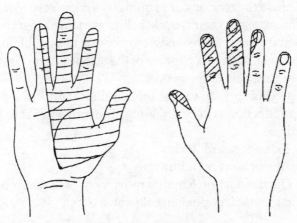

**Median nerve palsy,
sensory loss, wasting of thenar muscles**

Move

1. Movements of the fingers and thumb
2. Movements of the wrist
3. Power

Movements of the fingers and thumb

The movements of the fingers should be assessed together and then individually, as necessary. The patient should be asked to make a fist, and the grip felt for strength.

The metacarpo-phalangeal joints are assessed as well as the interphalangeal joints. Flexion at the distal phalanx is carried out by flexor profundus and at the middle phalanx by flexor superficialis. Flexor profundus is assessed by flexion of the distal interphalangeal joint of the fingers.

Flexor superficialis is tested by putting the profundus out of action by extending the fingers other than the one being assessed. The ability to flex the middle phalanx then signifies an intact superficialis tendon to that finger. This is because the tendons of profundus divide very low in the forearm and their muscle bellies are joined together.

Remember that weakness may be due to a problem in the muscle such as a rupture of the extensor tendon, or due to paralysis of the nerves.

The thumb is the most mobile digit, and impaired thumb function is very disabling. The movements to be tested are:

1. Extension and flexion
2. Abduction and adduction
3. Circumduction (circular movement of the thumb at the first metacarpophalangeal joint)

Hand and Wrist Examination

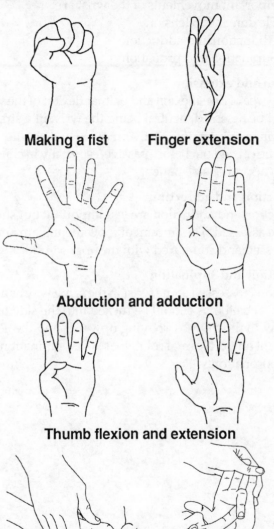

Making a fist   **Finger extension**

Abduction and adduction

Thumb flexion and extension

Flexor profundus   **Flexor superficialis**

Movements of the wrist

The important movements of the wrist are:
1. Flexion and extension
2. Abduction and adduction
3. Supination and pronation

Flexion and extension

The degree of dorsiflexion and palmar flexion of the wrist should be assessed, neutral being the wrist in a straight position, as illustrated. Active movements should normally be carried out before passive, especially in children and in apprehensive patients.

Abduction and adduction

Abduction and adduction are less important but should also be assessed. The amount of movement from neutral is assessed and compared with the opposite side.

Pronation and supination

Rotation is assessed at the wrist in the same way as at the elbow. The elbows should be tucked into the side of the body with the thumbs pointing upwards and the elbow at a right angle. Normal rotation is 90° of supination and 90° of pronation.

Hand and Wrist Examination

Flexion and extension

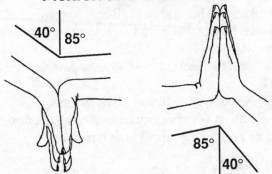

Abduction and adduction

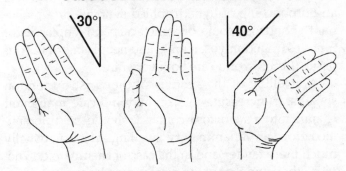

Pronation and supination

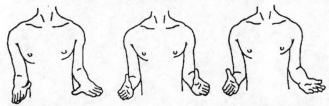

Limited on right   Neutral   Limited on right

Hand and Wrist Conditions

Congenital abnormalities

Deformities of a hand should always be compared to the other side. Bilateral deformity frequently signifies a congenital problem. These include:

Madelung's deformity — shortening or absence of the radius.

Polysyndactyly — fusion of the fingers.

Phocomelia — deficiency or shortening of one or more digits, or even of the whole limb (amelia).

Neoplasia

Neoplasms of the hand and wrist are uncommon. They include benign neoplasms such as a ganglion, which is an outpouching of hypertrophied synovia, or a malignant chondrosarcoma of a metacarpal. Neoplasms of muscles (rhabdomyosarcoma) and neoplasms of fibrous tissue (fibrosarcoma) are both very rare.

A swelling of the synovia of the wrist on tendon sheaths, if increasing in size, may indicate malignant change into a synoviosarcoma. It should be differentiated from an inflammatory swelling which is usually much more tender, and in the case of rheumatoid synovitis other evidence of the disease may be evident.

Hand and Wrist Conditions

Congenital abnormalities

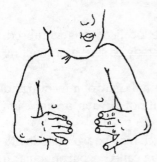

Madelung's deformity

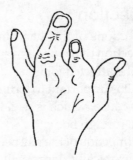

Polysyndactyly

Neoplasia

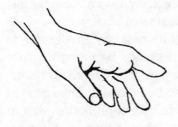

Enchondroma of index finger

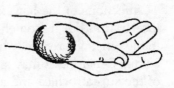

Chondrosarcoma of the first metacarpal

Trauma

Injuries to the hand and wrist are very common. Old fractures of the wrist are particularly common. There may be residual paralysis, scarring and ulceration as well as evidence of infection and sinuses.

Infection

Infections of the hand may be localised or generalised. Infection of the fingers or wrist may be seen as a swelling of the affected joint.

It is important to localise both the site of infection and the cause, which is usually, but not always, an abrasion or a foreign body.

Infection of the nail bed, which may be associated with a chronically damp nail bed, is called a paronychia. It usually causes redness and swelling at the base or along one edge of the nail.

An injury to the finger may cause considerable pain, particularly in the pulp of the finger. This infection may spread to the tendon sheath, and, if untreated, particularly in a flexor tendon, may cause infection of the individual or the common flexor sheath with considerable swelling in the palm and dorsum of the hand.

Infections of the hand and wrist are usually due to local trauma but are sometimes blood-borne, particularly in the wrist where it may be part of a generalised septicaemia. Other joints may also be involved. Enlargement of the supratrochlea and axillary lymph nodes should be looked for, as should a focus of primary infection such as the throat or genitourinary tract.

Hand and Wrist Conditions

Trauma

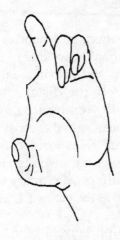

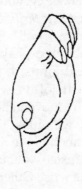

Amputation

Division of extensor digitorum tendons

Infection

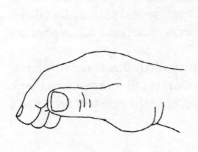

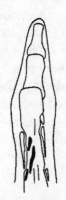

Swollen hand due to infection

X-ray appearance of osteomyelitis

Arthritis

Arthritis may be subdivided as:

1. Autoimmune eg. rheumatoid arthritis
2. Degenerative eg. osteoarthritis
3. Metabolic eg. gout

Rheumatoid arthritis commonly affects both hands and wrists symmetrically. There is normally swelling of the wrist, metacarpo-phalangeal joints and proximal inter-phalangeal joints, but only rarely the distal inter-phalangeal joints with warmth, tenderness and limitation of movement. In the latter stages there may be deformity with ulnar deviation and palmar dislocation or subluxation of the metacarpo-phalangeal joints, rupture of the extensor tendons and stiffness, deformity and pain in the wrist. Other joints such as the elbows, knees, ankles and feet are often involved.

In *osteoarthritis*, the distal interphalangeal joints are commonly affected (Heberden's nodes). This is in contrast to rheumatoid arthritis.

Miscellaneous conditions

Many other conditions affect the wrist and hand. These include Dupuytren's contracture and skin malignancies such as squamous cell carcinoma, basal cell carcinoma and melanoma.

Paralysis of the hand may occur due to nerve injuries (impaired sensation) or poliomyelitis (normal sensation), and this is discussed in detail in the relevant sections of this book.

Hand and Wrist Conditions

Arthritis

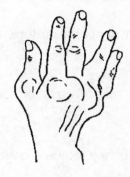

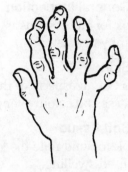

Rheumatoid arthritis   **Osteoarthritis**

Miscellaneous

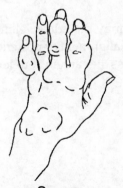

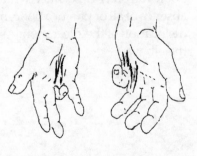

**Severe
tophaceous gout**   **Dupuytren's contracture**

Elbow and Forearm Examination

Look

1. General inspection
Look for any obvious asymmetry, abnormal posture, deformity or wasting.

2. Skin
Look at all aspects of the elbow and forearm for scars, sinuses and colour changes.

3. Soft tissue
Look for, and note the location of any localised or generalised swelling.

Localised swelling may be due to an enlarged olecranon bursa, rheumatoid nodules, gouty tophi or arise from the underlying bone.

General swelling may be due to infection or trauma.

Look for any wasting of the forearm muscles.

4. Bone and joint
Look for bony deformity which may include swelling, absence of all or part of a bone, malalignment or posterior dislocation of the olecranon. Assess the carrying angle of the elbow.

Elbow and Forearm Examination

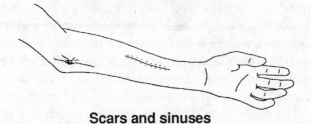

Scars and sinuses

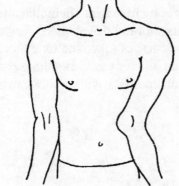

Cubitus valgus

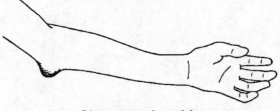

Olecranon bursitis

Feel

The elbow should be felt carefully for tender areas which usually gives a clue to the diagnosis. Tenderness over the lateral epicondyle itself may indicate a tennis elbow. Tenderness over the head of the radius may signify a fracture. Tenderness in the extensor muscles themselves *below* the lateral epicondyle may be associated with cervical spondylosis. The opposite side should always be compared, exerting the same amount of pressure.

The elbow should be palpated for warmth and, if indicated, for any sensory abnormalities.

Any swellings or deformities should be gently palpated to determine their consistency and whether they are soft tissue or bony in origin. Their attachments, margins and contents should be evaluated. Fluctuation and pulsation should also be looked for. One should attempt to transilluminate all soft tissue swellings, especially if soft, as ganglia and lipomata, will usually transilluminate.

Elbow and Forearm Examination

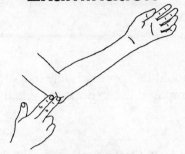

**Medial aspect,
tender, thickened ulnar nerve**

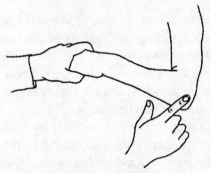

**Lateral aspect,
site of tenderness of a tennis elbow**

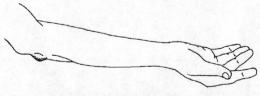

Rheumatoid nodules

Move

Elbow movements which should be examined are:
1. Flexion
2. Extension
3. Rotation

Flexion

Full flexion should be approximately 150°–160°. It should always be compared to the opposite side if there is any limitation.

Extension

Full extension is 0°. Occasionally the elbow may hyper-extend.

Rotation

Rotation of the forearm at the elbow is assessed by having both elbows close to the sides of the body with the thumbs facing upwards and the elbow flexed to approximately 90°. Pronation and supination of the two sides are compared. These should normally be 90° of pronation and 90° of supination.

Rotation may be limited, not only by elbow joint conditions including arthritis, infection and trauma but also by injury to the lower radio-ulnar joint. Deformity of either the radius or ulna due to a fracture, Paget's disease or other causes will also limit rotation.

Elbow and Forearm Examination

Flexion and Extension

Movement — 0°
to 130°

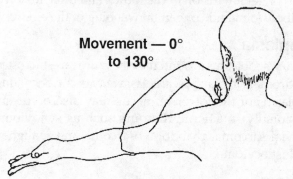

Rotation

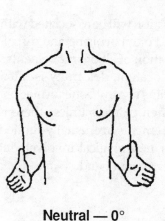

Neutral — 0°

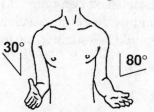

20°

90°

Pronation limited on right

30°

80°

Supination limited on right

Elbow and Forearm Conditions

Congenital abnormalities

Congenital elbow conditions are uncommon. They include congenital fusion of the radius and ulna, fusion of the elbow joint and congenital webbing of the elbow.

Neoplasia

Primary neoplasms around the elbow are rare, but osteochondromata in diaphyseal aclasia may occur. Secondary neoplasms of the lower humerus may also occur and occasionally soft tissue tumours such as synovioma, synovial sarcoma, rhabdomyosarcoma and malignant fibrohistiocytoma.

Trauma

A fracture or dislocation of the lower humerus or of the olecranon or head of the radius can cause deformity or swelling of the elbow.

A recent fracture or dislocation will be associated with pain, swelling, deformity and often bruising and discolouration. There will be limitation of elbow movements.

In an old fracture or dislocation, deformity is often present and there may be callus or new bone formation. The actual fracture site is often painless unless there is established non-union. Movements are usually limited and evidence of vascular or neurological involvement should be sought in the forearm and hand.

Elbow and Forearm Conditions

Congenital abnormalities

Neoplasia

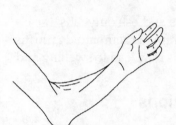

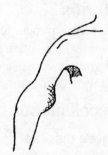

Webbing

Malignant fibrohistiocytoma

Trauma

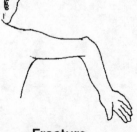

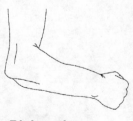

Fracture

Dislocation

Infection

Infection of the elbow joint may be associated with a compound fracture of the radius, ulna or lower humerus, or pyogenic arthritis (haematogenous spread or infection from an infected bursa). The whole elbow is often swollen and there may be redness and discharging sinuses.

Arthritis

Apart from pyogenic arthritis and osteomyelitis, the elbow may be swollen and painful in rheumatoid arthritis and gout. Severe osteoarthritis may lead to swelling and limitation of movement.

Miscellaneous conditions

Paget's disease

Paget's disease may be localised or generalised and often causes thickening and bowing of the radius or ulna. In the later stages the bone may be tender but usually it is merely deformed and slightly warmer than the opposite side, which must always be compared.

Elbow and Forearm Conditions

Infection

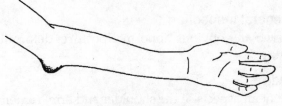

Olecranon bursitis

Arthritis

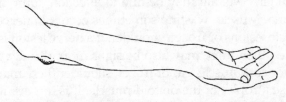

Rheumatoid nodules (extensor surfaces)

Paget's disease

Enlargement, bowing and elongation of radius

Shoulder and Humerus Examination

Look

1. General inspection

Observe any obvious abnormal posture, deformity or wasting.

2. Skin

Look at all aspects of the shoulder and arm, remembering the axilla and noting scars, sinuses or colour changes.

3. Soft tissues

Compare both shoulders looking for local or generalised swelling or change in muscle mass in the affected shoulder. Swelling may be due to infection, tumour or trauma. Muscle wasting sometimes occurs in nerve or muscle lesions or frozen shoulder. If a nerve lesion is involved then there may also be signs more distally. In a rotator cuff muscle tear or frozen shoulder there may be disuse atrophy of the deltoid muscle. It is important to look at wasting from the back, sides and front and to compare the two sides.

4. Bone and joint

Look at the anterior and posterior aspects of the shoulders to note symmetry, size and position of the clavicles and scapulae. Look for swelling in the antero-medial apect of the shoulder which may indicate anterior dislocation. Prominence of the lateral end of the clavicle may indicate subluxation or dislocation of the acromio-clavicular joint. Similarly, prominence of the medial end may indicate a past injury to the sterno-clavicular joint, clavicle and occasionally, tumour or infection.

Shoulder and Humerus Examination

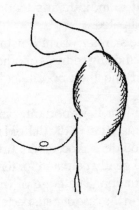

Soft tissue swelling

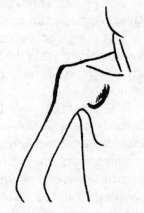

Anterior dislocation

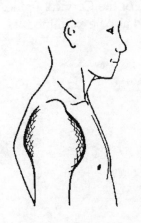

Osteosarcoma

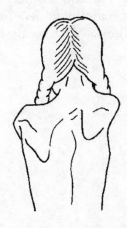

Sprengel's shoulder

Feel

After the shoulder has been inspected it should be systematically palpated.

The patient should be asked to indicate any tender areas which should be gently palpated.

The examiner should feel the skin for warmth using the dorsal surface of the fingers, and any redness or other discolouration should be noted and the opposite side compared.

The sensation over the shoulder is important, particularly the sensation over the insertion of the deltoid if a fracture or dislocation of the shoulder has occurred. Any swelling should be carefully and gently palpated for tenderness, consistency and fluctuation. The edge of the swelling should be felt carefully. In the case of a suspected infection or neoplastic lesion, regional lymph nodes, both in the axilla and the neck should be carefully palpated.

No examination of the shoulder is complete without a systematic examination of the neck. This is discussed specifically under, 'Examination of the Cervical Spine.' The distal part of the limb should also be examined.

Shoulder and Humerus Examination

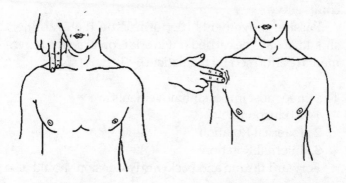

Clavicle   **Glenohumeral joint**

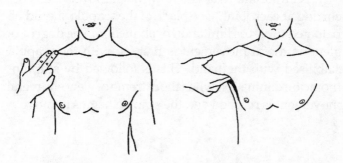

Tenderness   **Upper humeral shaft**

Move

In a child or apprehensive patient, the patient should be asked to move the arm gently outwards to gain confidence (active movements) before passive movements are commenced.

Passive movements (performed by the examiner) should always be carried out in addition to active movements (performed by the patient).

The three most important movements are:
1. Abduction
2. External Rotation
3. Internal Rotation

Forward flexion and backward extension should also be assessed.

Abduction

Normally 90° of abduction occurs at the gleno-humeral joint and 90° at the scapulothoracic, a total of 180°.

It is important to assess how much movement is occurring at each joint. The blade of the scapula should be palpated to assess limitation of abduction. The degree of gleno-humeral movement is first felt with the scapula stabilised with the hand. This is followed by scapulothoracic examination when the extreme of gleno-humeral movement is reached and the scapula begins to move.

Shoulder and Humerus Examination

Abduction and Adduction

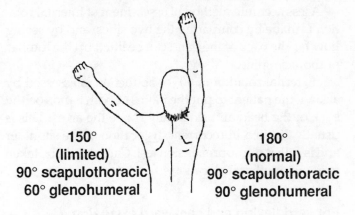

150°
(limited)
90° scapulothoracic
60° glenohumeral

180°
(normal)
90° scapulothoracic
90° glenohumeral

External Rotation   Internal Rotation

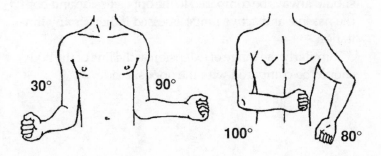

30°   90°

100°   80°

Rotation

The elbows are placed firmly into the sides, flexed at right angles, with the hands facing forwards. This is regarded as the neutral position. The degree of internal rotation and external rotation can then be assessed by comparing the two sides, as illustrated.

A less accurate method of assessment of internal rotation is made by comparing the two sides, and by seeing how far the back of the hand can be lifted up the lumbar or thoracic spine.

External rotation in 90° of abduction is assessed by asking the patient to put the palms of both hands on the back of the head and externally rotate the arms. This is usually limited in recurrent dislocation of the shoulder and is called the apprehension test. Care should be taken to avoid another dislocation.

Forward flexion and backward extension

The extent of forward flexion should be assessed with the arm lifted up in the line of the body. It may be possible to lift the arm fully to 180° in the line of body where it is limited in abduction due to the greater tuberosity of the humerus impinging on the acromion. Movement should always be compared to the opposite side and both the passive and active range assessed if there is any limitation.

Similarly the range of extension in the line of the body should be compared with the opposite side.

Shoulder and Humerus Conditions

Congenital abnormalities

These conditions are usually, but not always, bilateral. Examples include craniocleidodysostosis and Sprengel's shoulder.

Neoplasia

Primary tumours of the shoulder include osteogenic sarcoma, chondrosarcoma, aneurysmal bone cysts, and giant cell tumours. Other primary tumours may also affect the shoulder but are rare. Secondary deposits involving the shaft of the humerus are much more common than primary tumours.

Trauma

The most common injuries of the shoulder are dislocations and fractures. In dislocations, the head of the humerus is usually displaced anteriorly in the subcoracoid region. In a fracture the whole shoulder is swollen and often deformed. There may also be associated deltoid wasting after damage to the circumflex nerve. Other injuries around the shoulder joint include acromioclavicular subluxation and dislocation, and open wounds.

As well as the shoulder, it is important to examine the neck, chest and shaft of the humerus. The forearm and hand must also be carefully examined for weakness, sensory loss, vascular insufficiency or any other abnormalities and compared with the opposite side.

Shoulder and Humerus Conditions

Congenital abnormalities

Neoplasia

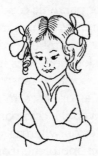

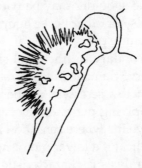

Craniocleidodysostosis

X-ray appearance of an osteogenic sarcoma

Trauma

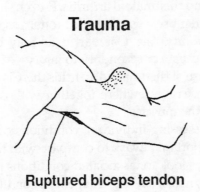

Ruptured biceps tendon

Infection

The shoulder may show considerable swelling, together with redness and pain. Infection may involve the entire shoulder or be localised.

Paralysis

The shoulder may be paralysed from a brachial plexus palsy or other nerve injuries. Other paralytic conditions include poliomyelitis and nerve injuries (which may be secondary to fractures) such as a circumflex (axillary) nerve damage in fractures and dislocations. It is important to assess whether there is any associated sensory loss implying peripheral nerve injury, as opposed to poliomyelitis where sensation is preserved. Flaccid paralysis indicates a lower motor neurone lesion whereas spastic paralysis is characteristic of upper motor neurone involvement.

Miscellaneous conditions

Other shoulder conditions include frozen shoulder, osteoarthritis and rheumatoid arthritis. Frozen shoulder may lead to rapid muscle wasting and is often associated with cervical spondylosis. Osteoarthritis may be primary (unknown cause) or secondary to injury.

In the case of rheumatoid arthritis there is usually evidence of disease elsewhere together with considerable wasting of the muscles.

When assessing individual conditions of the shoulder it is important always to compare with the opposite side. Always look for associated conditions providing a clue to diagnosis, such as congenital conditions, rheumatoid arthritis and trauma or infection.

Shoulder and Humerus Conditions

Infection

Paralysis

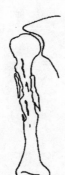

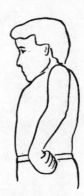

**X-ray appearance of
chronic osteomyelitis**

Erb's palsy

Miscellaneous conditions

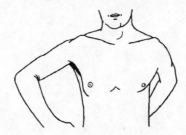

Frozen shoulder

Neurological Examination of the Upper Limb

Neurological assessment

1. Look
2. Feel — sensation
3. Move — tone

   power

   reflexes

   co-ordination

Brachial plexus lesions

1. Complete — C5 to T1
2. Upper — C5,6
3. Lower — C7,8,T1

Peripheral nerve lesions

1. Axillary
2. Median
3. Ulnar
4. Radial

Neurological Assessment

The upper limb may be paralysed by a lesion in the brain, the spinal cord or in the peripheral nerves. Assessment should include examination for sensory impairment i.e. light touch, pain and proprioception and motor involvement i.e. tone, power and reflexes.

Paralysis may be spastic (that is, an upper motor neurone due to cerebral or upper cervical cord involvement) or flaccid (that is, a lower motor neurone paralysis due to damage of the spinal roots, spinal cord or peripheral nerves). Upper and lower motor neurone damage sometimes co-exist.

Look

The affected limb must be compared with the opposite limb, together with the rest of the body, if indicated.

Inspection of the limb affected should include looking particularly for wasting, posture of the limb and deformity. Involuntary movements or a limb held in a flexed position, for instance, may indicate a spastic paralysis or a contracture. Muscle fasciculation, if present, should be noted. This is a sign of a lower motor neurone lesion. Lack of sweating and hair loss should be noted.

Feel

Muscle bulk and temperature changes should be compared by palpation of both upper limbs.

Sensation

The dermatomes of the upper limb are illustrated, but it should be noted that there is often considerable sensory overlap. Sensory testing should include light touch, pin-

Upper Limb Dermatomes

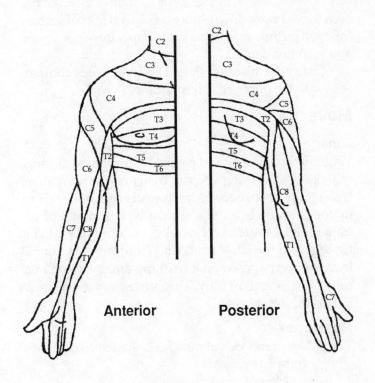

Anterior   Posterior

prick (pain), and proprioception, as a minimum for every patient with a possible neurological lesion.

Proprioception, or joint position sense is examined by holding the lateral aspects of the digit and passively dorsiflexing and extending it, while the patient, with eyes closed, nominates whether he or she thinks the digit has been moved up or down. More specialised tests of sensory function include examination of temperature perception and vibration sense.

Sensory examination should always include comparison with the opposite, 'normal' limb.

Move

Tone

The limb should be moved passively through its full range of motion, at varying speeds. Tone may be normal, increased, or decreased. Hypertonia is seen with upper motor neurone lesions, and may be pyramidal or extrapyramidal, the former typically producing 'clasp knife' rigidity, and the latter producing 'lead pipe' rigidity. A tremor superimposed on an extrapyramidal lesion may cause 'cog-wheel' rigidity. This is most commonly seen in Parkinson's disease.

Muscle power

The power of individual muscles is graded from 0 to 5:

0 — complete paralysis
1 — a flicker of movement only
2 — able to move when gravity is eliminated
3 — just able to move against gravity
4 — able to move against gravity with some resistance
5 — normal

Adding '1/2' or '+' signifies a power in between two grades. A detailed assessment of sensory deficit should

Muscle Power

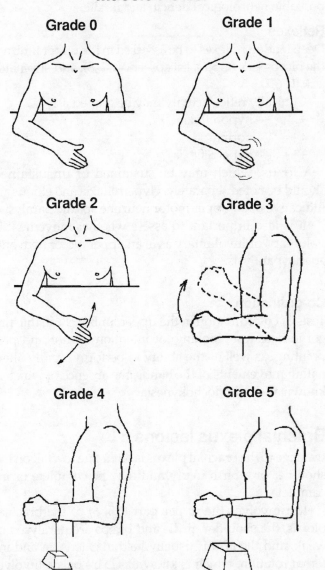

Grade 0

Grade 1

Grade 2

Grade 3

Grade 4

Grade 5

always be considered with motor power to assess the probable neurological deficit, and its site.

Reflexes

Deep tendon reflexes to be assessed in the upper limb are the biceps jerk (C 5,6), triceps jerk (C 7,8), and supinator jerk (C 6,7).

Clinically reflex activity may be graded as:

+   — hyporeflexia

++   — normal

+++   — hyperreflexia

Clonus, which may be sustained or unsustained should be noted separately. Hyperreflexia and clonus are indicative of an upper motor neurone spastic paralysis.

It is also important to assess whether movement is voluntary, or involuntary as in an upper motor neuronal spastic paralysis.

Co-ordination

Tests of co-ordination in the upper limb include the 'finger-to-nose test', looking for intention tremor and past pointing, as well as the ability to perform rapidly alternating movements of the hands, the absence of which is known as dysdiadochokynesia.

Brachial plexus lesions

Damage to the brachial plexus is often due to a fall on the shoulder or a birth injury and may be complete or incomplete.

If it involves the upper part (C5, 6) of the brachial plexus, the shoulder girdle and biceps are paralysed or weak, and the arm is usually held in extension and internal rotation, which is known as Erb's palsy. Involve-

Brachial Plexus Lesions

Birth injuries

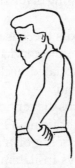 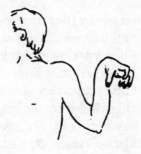

Erb's palsy   **Klumpke's palsy**

Trauma

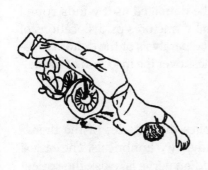 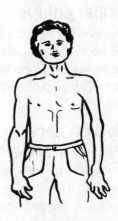

Fall on point of shoulder   **Flail arm**

ment of the lower brachial plexus (C 7, 8 and T 1) will cause paralysis of the triceps, forearm and small muscles of the hand. This is known as a Klumpke type of paralysis, and is less common.

In a complete palsy, the whole arm is paralysed and the only movement possible is shrugging of the shoulder carried out by the trapezius.

In all injuries of the brachial plexus there is sensory loss. It is important also to examine the cervical spine and the other three limbs, as an associated neck injury and other trauma are commonly found.

In high lesions of the brachial plexus the cervical sympathetic nerves may be involved, producing a Horner's syndrome. This is characterised by some or all of the following features (which are always ipsilateral to the lesion): ptosis ('dropped' lid), miosis (pupillary constriction), anhydrosis (lack of sweating), and enophthalmos.

Peripheral Nerve Lesions

Axillary nerve

The axillary nerve may be damaged as it winds round the neck of the humerus by fractures or dislocations of the shoulder. There will be paralysis of the deltoid muscle and an area of numbness over the insertion of the deltoid.

Median nerve

The median nerve supplies the muscles of the thenar eminence and also the radial two lumbricals. The easiest method of testing the median nerve is to ask the patient to abduct the thumb at *right* angles to the palm. Strength is then assessed and compared to that of the opposite side.

Median Nerve Lesions

Look

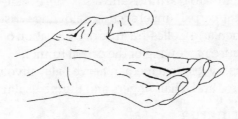

Thenar wasting

Feel

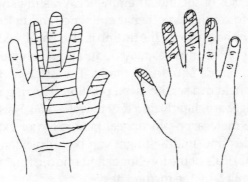

Move

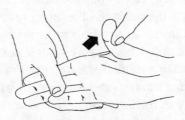

Thumb abduction

The median nerve is usually partially paralysed in a carpal tunnel syndrome. This occurs in situations where there is oedema in the carpal tunnel, such as in pregnancy, and rheumatoid arthritis and also where there is narrowing of the carpal tunnel such as following wrist fractures. In particular, a Colles' fracture or dislocation of the lunate may cause narrowing of the carpal tunnel.

Sensory loss in a median nerve palsy involves the radial three and a half fingers and thumb as illustrated.

Ulnar nerve

The ulnar nerve supplies all the small muscles of the hand, with the exception of the lateral two lumbricals and the muscles of the thenar eminence. Wasting should be looked for in the hypothenar eminence and in the inter-ossei. The adductor of the thumb is also paralysed. Gross wasting of the muscles may occur and a comparison of the two hands should be made. The affected hand is usually held in a semi-clawed position. The ring and the little finger are slightly flexed at the interphalangeal joints and the metacarpo-phalangeal joint is hyper-extended. The index and middle finger can be fully extended by the lumbricals of the forefinger and middle finger which are supplied by the median nerve.

In a high ulnar nerve lesion, the flexion deformity of the ring and little fingers may be much less. This is because the long flexors to the ring and little fingers are paralysed and cannot flex the ulnar two fingers. This phenomenon is called ulnar paradox, because a higher lesion produces less deformity than a more distal ulnar nerve lesion.

Other tests for ulnar nerve function include testing for the inability of the little finger to abduct against resistance and the inability to hold a card between the little

Ulnar Nerve Lesions

Look

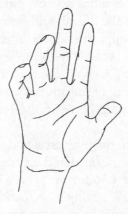

**Hypothenar and interosseous wasting together
with clawing of the ring and little fingers**

Feel — Sensation

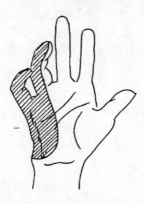

finger and ring finger as a result of paralysis of the interosseous muscles and lumbricals.

Froment's sign is a test of adductor pollicis. A card is held between the thumb and the forefingers of both hands, and the examiner pulls the card away while the patient resists. If the ulnar nerve is paralysed, the interphalangeal joint of the thumb will flex fully to hold the card, whilst on the opposite side the interphalangeal joint is extended. This is because the long flexor of the thumb is brought into play to hold the card to the forefinger. There is also wasting of the adductor pollicis and interossei in the web space between the 1st and 2nd metacarpals.

Paralysis of both the interossei and lumbricals of the 4th and 5th fingers means that the patient cannot hold a card between these two fingers. There is also weakness or complete paralysis of finger abduction.

Sensory disturbance in an ulnar nerve palsy involves one and a half fingers on the ulnar side of the hand as illustrated. It may also extend up the ulnar side of the lower forearm in high nerve palsies. In addition there may be a lack of sweating of the affected hand, which feels drier than normal. In long standing cases there will also be loss of hair, lack of skin wrinkling and a shiny appearance. These are known as trophic changes.

Ulnar Nerve Lesions

Move

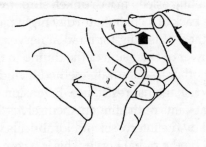

Abduction of little finger in line of palm

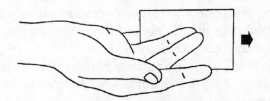

Testing finger adduction

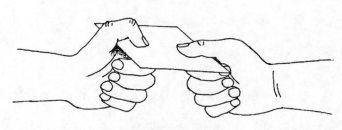

Froment's sign

Radial nerve

Radial nerve palsy is commonly caused by a fracture of the mid-shaft of the humerus. Other causes include pressure in the axilla by crutches that are too long (crutch palsy), and falling asleep in a drunken stupor with one's arm over the back of a chair (Saturday night palsy!). The quickest method of testing for a radial nerve palsy is to assess the power of extension of the thumb in the line of the palm. Another less accurate method includes extension of the wrist against resistance. Extension of the interphalangeal joints of the fingers themselves, however, is performed by the interossei and lumbricals which are not supplied by the radial nerve. This is a common trap for the unwary examiner and many radial nerve palsies have been missed as a result. A high lesion will result in a complete wrist drop while a low lesion, or one affecting the posterior interosseous nerve alone may affect dorsiflexion of the thumb and the fingers at the metacarpo-phalangeal joints alone.

The sensory loss in a radial nerve injury is a small area at the base of the thumb but this may extend to the back of the hand.

Radial Nerve Lesions

Look

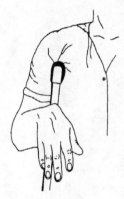

Wrist drop

Feel

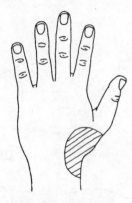

Sensory deficit

Move

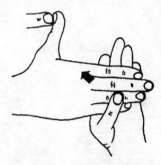

Testing thumb extension

Assessment of Peripheral Nerve Lesions — Summary

Power   Sensation

Median nerve

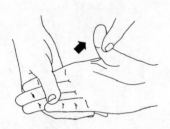
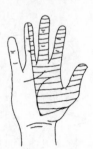

Ulnar nerve

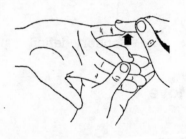
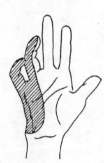

Radial nerve

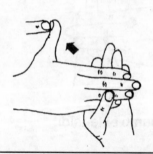
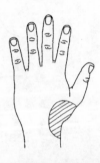

Chapter 3

Examination of the Spine

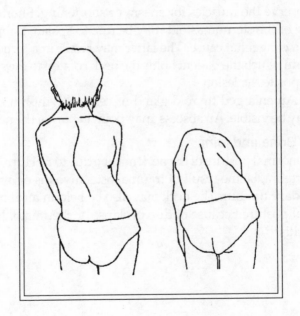

Cervical Spine Examination

Look

1. General inspection

Inspect the neck for any obvious swelling or deformity from the front, back and sides. The patient may also be in obvious pain.

2. Skin

Look for any evidence of scars, sinuses or colour change. There may be congenital webbing of the neck.

3. Soft tissue

Observe the muscles for spasm or shortening. Shortening of the sternomastoid may be due to spasm, trauma or a congenital cause. The latter may result in a torticollis, in which the patient holds the neck rotated to the side opposite the lesion.

An enlarged thyroid gland or cervical lymph nodes may be visible. An abscess may point in part of the neck.

4. Bone and joint

Abnormal posture of the neck may be due to fracture of a vertebra, be the result of trauma, osteomyelitis or a secondary tumour. The neck may also be held in an abnormal posture because of disc prolapse or rheumatoid arthritis.

Cervical Spine Examination

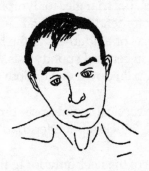

**Torticollis or 'wryneck' — may be
secondary to prolapsed disc**

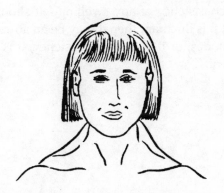

Congenital webbing of the neck

Feel

The neck should be felt for tenderness and swellings. The front of the neck should be felt for the thyroid, the anterior and posterior cervical triangles for lymph nodes, and the back of the neck for tender areas and swellings.

Localised areas of tenderness at the base of the neck may be present in cervical spondylosis. There may also be 'radiation' of pain down one or both arms to the fingers.

Classically in cervical spondylosis, three tender areas, representing the 'Huckstep tender triad', should be felt for. These are:

1. At the base of the neck anterior to the trapezius
2. Over the insertion of the deltoid
3. In the extensor mass of the forearm (not the origin of the extensors which usually suggests tennis elbow).

The consistency of any swelling felt should then be noted. If it is fluctuant then it may be an abscess, if firm, lymph nodes, or if of bony consistency, it is possibly a cervical rib.

Cervical Spine Examination

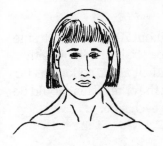

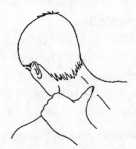

Prominence of cervical rib

Tenderness in base of neck — cervical spondylosis

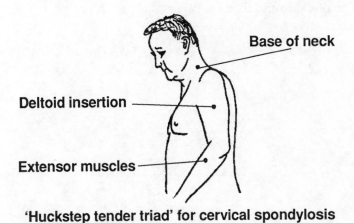

Base of neck

Deltoid insertion

Extensor muscles

'Huckstep tender triad' for cervical spondylosis

Move

The neck movements to be examined are:
1. Rotation
2. Flexion and extension
3. Lateral flexion

Rotation

Rotation should be equal, and about 70°–90° to each side as illustrated. The neck should be straight without either flexion or extension and the patient asked to look as far as possible to one side and then the other. This should be followed by passive rotation to each side.

Flexion and extension

Full forward flexion is present when the chin touches the chest. Full extension of at least 30° beyond the horizontal should be possible, and is usually greater in young people.

Lateral flexion

Lateral flexion should be at least 40° to each side. Again starting from the neutral position the head is tilted first to one side and then the other.

Cervical Spine Examination

Rotation

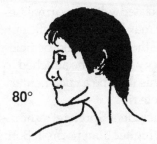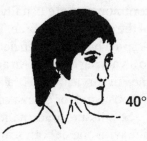

80°   40°

Flexion and extension

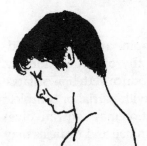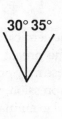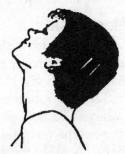

30° 35°

Lateral flexion

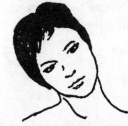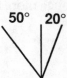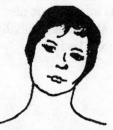

50° 20°

Cervical Spine Conditions

Congenital abnormalities

Congenital abnormalities of the cervical spine are not common and are usually associated with abnormalities of the cervical vertebrae. These may be fused or deficient. A spina bifida is a deficiency of the laminae and pedicles to a varying degree. An accessory rib may be attached to the 7th cervical vertebra and this may be a rudimentary fibrous band, or even a complete rib.

Soft tissue abnormalities include a Sprengel's shoulder, with one or both scapulae higher than normal. Both this and congenital webbing of the neck may be associated with cervical vertebral abnormalities or other congenital abnormalities such as cardiac defects.

Neoplasia

Most neoplasms of the cervical spine are due to secondary deposits from the breast, thyroid, lung, kidney, prostate or cervix. These may produce vertebral collapse and cord or root compression, with partial or complete paralysis. Radiological examination may show involvement of the vertebral bodies; laminae and pedicles may be involved but the disc spaces are usually spared. Neurofibromata of the spinal roots may also cause nerve or spinal cord compression. This is in contradistinction to an infection or disc degeneration where the intervertebral discs are initially much more involved than the vertebral bodies.

Cervical Spine Conditions

Congenital abnormalities

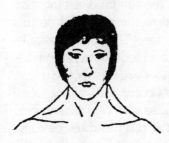

Congenital webbing of the neck

Neoplasia

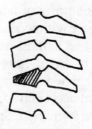

X-ray appearance of a secondary deposit

Trauma

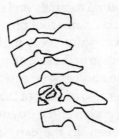

X-ray appearance of a fracture dislocation

Trauma

There may be severe root or spinal cord compression following dislocation or fracture dislocation of the cervical vertebrae, including the odontoid process of C2.

Infection

Infection of the cervical spine usually involves the disc spaces, and may later spread to the vertebral bodies (compare with secondary tumours). The onset is usually acute, and in most cases due to a blood borne staphylococcal infection. Infection by other organisms, including the tubercle bacillus, may also occur but with a more gradual onset and sometimes also with retropharyngeal abscess formation. Spasm of the cervical muscles commonly results in marked limitation of neck movements, and cord compression may also occur.

Arthritis

Osteoarthritis and cervical spondylosis

Degeneration of the disc spaces, particularly C4/5 and C5/6, is common, and is often associated with narrowing of the intervertebral foramen and osteophyte formation. This, in turn, may cause root pressure on the C5 and 6 roots on one or both sides. Neck movements are limited, particularly rotation to the side affected, lateral flexion to the opposite side and neck extension. The 'Huckstep tender triad' (tenderness at: base of the neck, insertion of the deltoid muscle and over the extensor muscles of the forearm) is often seen. In the early stages of cervical spondylosis X-rays may appear normal.

Cervical Spine Conditions

Infection

Arthritis

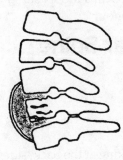

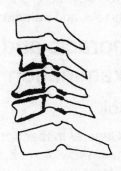

**X-ray appearance of
tuberculosis with a
'cold' abscess**

**X-ray appearance of
cervical spondylosis**

Miscellaneous conditions

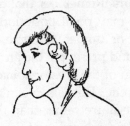

**Rheumatoid arthritis:
limited rotation with muscle spasm**

Rheumatoid arthritis and other conditions

Rheumatoid arthritis can cause considerable pain and stiffness of the cervical spine. It may lead to subluxation and dislocation of the vertebrae due to softening of the ligaments. Nerve root and spinal cord compression may also occur. Other conditions of the neck include spasmodic torticollis, and a sternomastoid 'tumour'.

Thoracic and Lumbar Spine Examination

Look

1. General inspection

Note any obvious abnormality, looking at the back, sides and front of the patient.

2. Skin

Look for scars, sinuses or colour change. Note the presence of a hair tuft, discolouration or dimpling at the base of the spine indicating a spina bifida.

3. Soft tissue

Look for any swellings which may be due to infection, trauma, or tumours. Remember that an abscess in the vertebral column may point posteriorly or, if affecting the lower thoracic or lumbar vertebrae, may track down the psoas sheath and present in the groin.

Look for spasm of the erector spinae muscles on either side of the spine. This is sometimes a cause of abnormal spinal curvature rather than the presence of a defect in the vertebral column itself. Scoliosis may be due to muscle spasm, paralysis or to a congenital or idiopathic scoliosis.

Thoracic and Lumbar Spine Examination

Kyphoscoliosis

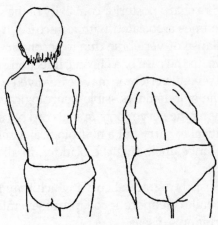

Idiopathic kyphoscoliosis

Kyphosis

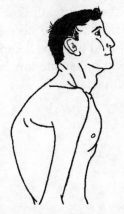

4. Bone and joint

Look from the posterior and lateral aspects of the patient for any increase or decrease in spinal curvature i.e. scoliosis or kyphosis.

Kyphos and kyphosis

A kyphos is a sharp posterior convexity of the spinal column sometimes associated with a fracture. It may also follow collapse of vertebrae due to secondary deposits or infection. In the case of a chronic infection such as tuberculosis several vertebrae may be involved with shortening of the spine and possible neurological compression involving the nerve roots, spinal cord or corda equina. It is critical to carry out a neurological assessment of the lower limbs, including the bladder, in all these patients.

A kyphosis is a gradual curve which may be due to paralysis, senile osteoporotic collapse of several vertebrae or Scheuermann's disease.

Lordosis

A lordosis is a posterior concavity of the spinal column, often in the lumbar region. It may be associated with low back pain, paralysis or spondylolisthesis. In pregnancy a compensatory lordosis may be necessary to maintain balance. This, combined with the lax spinal ligaments in later pregnancy, may potentiate low back strain sometimes associated with sciatica.

Thoracic and Lumbar Spine

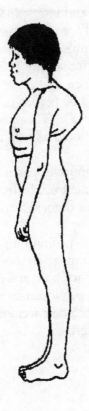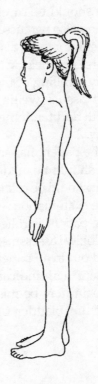

Thoracic kyphos

Excessive lumbar lordosis

Feel

After inspection, the spine should be palpated gently. It is important to feel the spine for tender areas, both in the midline and laterally.

The vertebral spinous processes and interspinal ligaments should be carefully palpated for tenderness and gaps and also percussed gently. The muscles on each side of the spine should also be palpated for spasm. This may be worse on one side than on the other.

Any swelling of the spine should be palpated. Bony or soft tissue swelling or an abscess may be present. Warmth and tenderness should be noted as well as deformity.

If the patient has severe pain or muscle spasm no attempt should be made to sit the patient up. Instead the patient should be rolled over to one or other side to carry out the examination.

The patient is rolled into a supine position for a full neurological assessment. A rectal examination should be carried out in all patients with low back pain and sciatica, where this is indicated; otherwise pelvic causes of low back pain may be missed. These include carcinoma of the rectum, bladder, prostate and uterus.

Thoracic and Lumbar Spine Examination

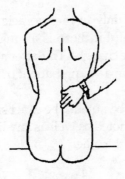

Palpate

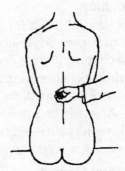

Percuss gently for tenderness

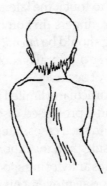

Feel for muscle spasm

Move

The three main movements of the thoracic and lumbar spine are:

1. Rotation
2. Lateral flexion
3. Flexion and extension

Rotation

Rotation of the spine occurs mainly in the thoracic region. It may be limited or painful if there is an injury, infection, tumour or degenerative changes. The latter may include Scheuermann's disease in a young patient or osteoarthritis in an older patient.

Any pain on rotation should be noted. The exact spot where the pain is felt should be noted as well as any limitation of rotation to one side or the other.

Lateral Flexion

Lateral flexion of the spine occurs mainly in the lumbar region. The patient should be asked to bend first to one side and then to the other.

The arms must be kept close to the body and the patient should attempt to touch the lateral side of the knee with the outstretched fingers first on one side and then on the other. Bending should be *lateral*, not forward. Any difference in the degree of lateral flexion can then be noted with a fair degree of accuracy.

Lateral flexion is particularly limited in conditions such as low back strain and a prolapsed disc in the lumbar or lumbo-sacral region. In such cases, lateral flexion is often more limited to one side than the other.

In conditions such as ankylosing spondylitis, infections and fractures, however, all movements may be restricted.

Thoracic and Lumbar Spine Examination

Rotation — thoracic spine

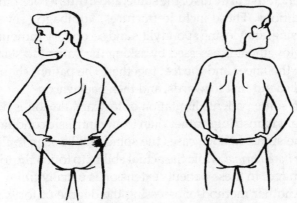

Limited rotation to right

Lateral flexion — lumbar spine

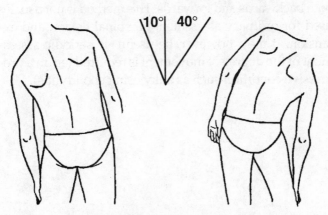

10° 40°

Limited lateral flexion to left

Flexion and extension

Flexion and extension occur both in the lumbar region and the hips, but more so in the hips.

Forward flexion and backward extension are both limited in prolapse of an intervertebral disc, in severe degenerative arthritis of the spine, and in numerous other conditions. These include fractures, 'lumbago', severe bruising, ankylosing spondylitis and secondary tumours.

Movement is assessed by asking the patient to stand with the knees and the feet together. The patient should *gently* bend first forwards, and then backwards.

In some patients limitation of forward flexion is due to tight hamstrings rather than to any intrinsic condition of the spine. In such cases the spine will be seen to flex *more than normal* while the actual ability to touch the toes is limited. In these patients extension is usually full.

Another method of assessing the degree of forward flexion is to mark two points in the upper and lower parts of the thoracic and lumbar spine respectively. The distance between the points is measured as the patient bends both backwards and forwards. This method is not usually used for ordinary assessment of spinal flexion and extension. It may, however, be useful if periodic assessment of the degree of movement is required (eg. in a progressive condition such as ankylosing spondylitis).

Thoracic and Lumbar Spine Examination

Flexion — lumbar spine and hips

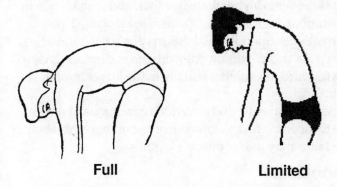

Full

Limited

Extension — lumbar spine and hips

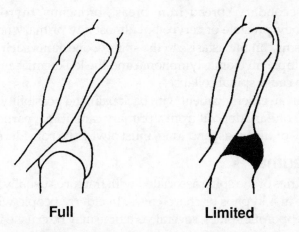

Full

Limited

Thoracic and Lumbar Spine Conditions

Congenital abnormalities

Congenital conditions of the thoracic and lumbar spine are uncommon. They include Sprengel shoulder, where one shoulder is higher than the other, and spina bifida in the lumbar region with or without associated meningomyelocele. Spondylolisthesis may be congenital or acquired. In this condition one vertebra is displaced, usually forward, on another usually in the lower lumbar region.

Scoliosis may be due to various conditions. It may be due to incomplete development of one or more vertebrae. The latter may also produce a kyphos.

Neoplasia

Primary spinal neoplasms are rare. Secondary deposits, on the other hand, are common and may cause collapse of one or more vertebrae.They are most commonly due to secondary spread from breast, bronchus, thyroid, kidney, prostate or cervix, but almost any primary neoplasms can metastasise to the spine. Conditions such as multiple myeloma, lymphoma and the leukaemias may also cause spinal collapse.

In an elderly patient with back pain, the possibility of a secondary deposit from a primary carcinoma, particularly of the breast and lung, must always be considered.

Trauma

Injuries of the spine associated with fractures usually result in a kyphos or sharp curve. In elderly people with osteoporotic spines, several vertebrae may be crushed at

Thoracic and Lumbar Spine Conditions

Congenital abnormalities

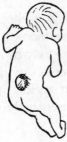

Spina bifida with meningomyelocele

Neoplasia

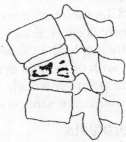

X-ray appearance of spinal metastasis producing a kyphos

Trauma

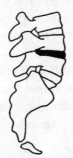

X-ray appearance of posterior disc prolapse at L4/5

one time, particularly in the thoracic region, often resulting in a smooth kyphosis.

Infection

Infections of the spine are uncommon. They include blood borne infections which are often seen in patients who are in poor health such as drug addicts. Infections of the disc spaces may follow lumbar puncture or occasionally a spinal operation.

Chronic infections of the spine include brucellosis and tuberculosis. A disc and two adjoining vertebrae are initially involved. In time several vertebrae may be affected, with or without evidence of an abscess. An abscess may point posteriorly or in the lumbar region. It may also track down the psoas sheath and present in the groin.

Paralysis

Paralysis of the spine sometimes leads to a scoliosis and, if it is severe, to a kypho-scoliosis with prominence of the ribs on one side due to rotation of the vertebrae.

In the past the most common paralytic disorder causing scoliosis was poliomyelitis. This could lead to a scoliosis by producing asymmetrical spinal muscle paralysis. In a child this could be corrected by lifting the shoulders and upper body. In older patients it is more difficult to correct completely due to fibrosis of the muscles and fascia.

Other paralytic conditions include a scoliosis associated with injury to the spinal cord, or associated with cerebral conditions including brain tumours, cerebral palsy, stroke and head injuries.

Thoracic and Lumbar Spine Conditions

Infection

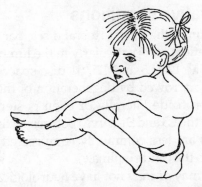

Tuberculous kyphos with 'cold' abscess

Idiopathic conditions

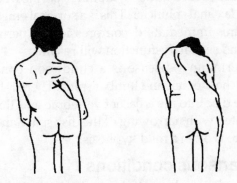

Kyphoscoliosis demonstrated on forward flexion

Idiopathic conditions

This is a scoliosis of unknown aetiology which usually arises in childhood. It is maintained and is exacerbated on forward flexion, unlike a scoliosis due to a short leg which usually disappears on forward flexion.

Degenerative conditions

Degeneration of the intervertebral discs, particularly in the older patient and particularly in the lumbar spine is common. The L4/L5 and L5/S1 disc spaces are most likely to be narrowed by degeneration of the disc. The disc may protrude laterally or even posteriorly with pressure on the L5 and S1 nerve roots respectively. Other nerve roots are less commonly compressed and occasionally also the cauda equina.

Patients may or may not have neurological signs associated with this. Signs of disc prolapse include limitation of straight leg raising and diminished or absent reflexes and sensory disturbances in the lower limbs. A central disc prolapse may press on the cauda equina and be associated with bladder symptoms, perineal sensory loss and a lax anal sphincter. This is a surgical emergency and requires immediate decompression or permanent bladder and sexual dysfunction will result.

Scheuermann's disease is a childhood condition involving the thoracic and lumbar spine. There is herniation of the disc into the adjacent vertebrae and this may be associated with narrowing of the disc space and back pain. There is often a mild kyphosis.

Miscellaneous conditions

These include the rheumatoid group of diseases affecting mainly the spine initially, such as ankylosing spondylitis, through to rheumatoid arthritis where the

Thoracic and Lumbar Spine Conditions

Degenerative conditions

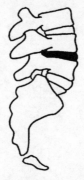

X-ray appearance of disc degeneration and prolapse; usually L4/L5 or L5/S1

Miscellaneous conditions

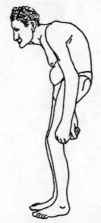

Ankylosing spondylitis

spine is often only affected late in the disease. The sacro-iliac joints may be involved early in ankylosing spondy-litis, and late in rheumatoid arthritis.

Chapter 4

Examination of the Lower Limb

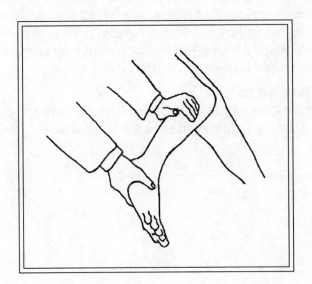

Lower Limb Examination

Gait

The patient should be examined walking, preferably with and without shoes. Abnormal gait includes:

1. Antalgic gait
2. Short leg gait
3. Paralytic gait
4. Trendelenburg gait
5. Stiff leg gait
6. Other

Antalgic gait

This is the gait associated with a painful leg or foot. The patient walks with a minimum of weight on the painful side and will try to take the weight back to the normal side as quickly as possible. The patient may grimace as the weight is taken on the painful side.

Short leg gait

In the short leg gait the patient will dip down on the short leg during weight bearing on the affected side.

Lower Limb Examination

Examining gait

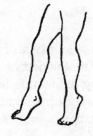

Walking on toes

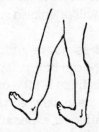

Walking on heels

Abnormal types of gait

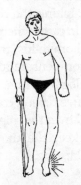

Antalgic gait

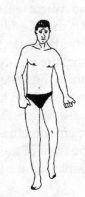

Short leg gait

Paralytic gait

Paralytic gait occurs when one or both legs are paralysed. The paralysis may be spastic or flaccid.

Spastic gait occurs in conditions such as cerebral palsy, following a stroke, cerebral tumour, skull fracture or infection in the brain, cervical or thoracic spine. The common factor is an upper motor neurone injury. The patient will often also walk with a flexed hip, knee and ankle.

The legs may be adducted and a scissor type of gait is typical of cerebral palsy. In upper motor neurone type paralysis there is little or no wasting of the muscles and the legs are usually equal in length. The upper limb may also be affected, especially in cerebral palsy or stroke. All four limbs may also be affected.

In a *flaccid paralytic* gait there are different degrees of weakness between individual joints and muscles. This is unlike the spastic gait when the whole of one or both lower limbs tends to be equally paralysed.

In the flaccid gait due to a foot drop, such as occurs with common peroneal and anterior tibial muscle paralysis, the patient will walk dragging the toe. Alternatively, the step may be high to avoid catching the toe on the ground as the leg swings forward. In cases where the knee extensors are paralysed, as in poliomyelitis, the patient may brace the knee in order to compensate for a weak knee extensor and to prevent the leg buckling.

In cases where there is also a knee flexion contracture the patient sometimes uses a hand over the thigh to support the front of the thigh and to keep the knee straight as possible and the knee from collapsing.

Lower Limb Examination

Abnormal types of gait

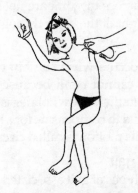

**Paralytic gait; scissor gait
secondary to cerebral palsy**

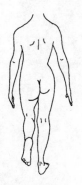

Trendelenburg gait

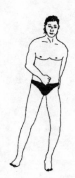

Stiff leg gait

Trendelenburg gait

If the hip is painful, weak, dislocated or fractured, its stability is affected. As a result the pelvis tilts down to the opposite side instead of tilting up when walking. This is because either the fulcrum of the joint is deficient or the muscles acting across the joint are not strong enough to stabilise the weight of the body through the hip joint.

Stiff leg gait

A stiff leg gait occurs when the hip or knee has been arthrodesed or cannot bend because of pain, limited movement or splinting. The whole leg is swung outwards to clear the ground to compensate for a hip or knee which cannot bend. This motion is called circumduction.

Other types of gait

There are other types of gait associated with a deformity or stiffness. A combined type of gait is sometimes seen when a short leg combined with a paralytic leg and antalgic gait all occur in the same patient.

Leg Shortening

Classification

Type

    True (real) shortening

    Apparent shortening

    Combined true and apparent

Site

    Above knee

    Below knee

    Ankle and foot

True shortening

Real shortening is present when the affected leg is *actually shorter* in *overall length* than the opposite limb. It is measured with the *pelvis square* or level if possible. The measurement is taken from the anterior superior iliac spine to the medial malleolus with the legs and the sole of the foot in the same position. This measurement should then be extended down to the *bottom of the heel* with the ankle in the neutral position. It is compared to the length of the opposite leg in the same position.

If there is a fixed abduction, adduction or flexion deformity of one hip which cannot be corrected, the opposite leg should be abducted, adducted or flexed to the *same* position before the measurement is taken. If the knee is in fixed flexion the opposite knee should be flexed to the same position before measurement. Similarly, if the ankle is in equinus or in a deformed position the opposite ankle or foot must be placed as near as possible in the same position before measurement.

True or real shortening is the *real* difference between the length of the legs. *Apparent* shortening is the shortening as it appears to the patient.

In assessing the amount of raise on the shoe required to compensate for the shortening, the *apparent*, rather than the *real* shortening must be taken into account. The patient with a fixed adduction deformity of hip or flexion contracture of knee, will still walk with these deformities until they have been corrected. The patient is only concerned with the distance of the sole of the foot from the floor when walking.

Leg Shortening

Real shortening   Apparent shortening

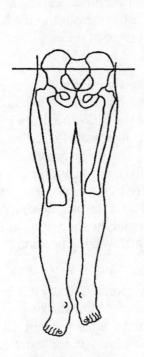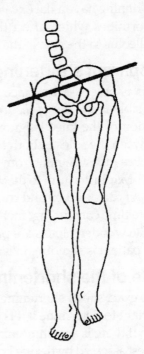

**Pelvis squared
Measure from ASIS to
medial malleolus and
sole of foot. Adduct
opposite leg if fixed
adduction**

**Pelvis tilted
Measure from
xiphisternum to
medial malleolus and
sole of foot**

Unfortunately most text books still describe measurement of the leg from the anterior superior iliac spine to the medial malleolus of the ankle instead of to the bottom of the sole of the foot. People do not walk on the medial malleolus but on the sole of the foot! Many patients with shortening have a flat or cavus foot or other heel and foot deformities which affect the distance from the medial malleolus to the sole of the foot on each side.

Apparent shortening

This is assessed by placing the two limbs as near as possible *in the line of the trunk*. Any tilt of the pelvis or flexion of the knee is ignored. The difference in height between the soles of both feet is then assessed. Alternatively a measurement from the pubic symphysis, umbilicus or xiphisternum to the medial malleoli *and the soles of the feet* can be taken and compared. A more accurate, but more time consuming, method is for the patient to stand while wooden blocks are put under the shorter leg until the patient is standing in a normal walking position.

Site of the shortening

The exact site of shortening is important. Firstly it is important to determine if it is above or below the knee and also if there is any shortening in the ankle and foot. This is best assessed by flexing both knees to 90°, as illustrated.

Leg Shortening

Site of shortening

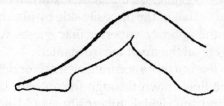

Normal

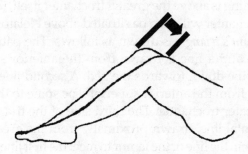

Above the knee

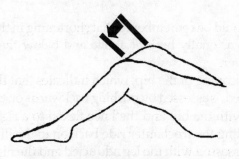

Below the knee

Shortening above the knee

In assessing shortening above the knee it is important to decide whether it occurs above the greater trochanter, or below the trochanter in the femoral shaft itself. The elevation of the trochanter on the shorter side can be quickly compared to that of the opposite side by placing one's thumbs on the anterior superior iliac spines with the middle fingers on the tip of the trochanters.

Nelaton's line is a more accurate method for determining this. The line drawn through the anterior superior iliac spine and the ischial tuberosity should normally pass through the top of the greater trochanter. If the shortening is above the greater trochanter itself, the tip of the trochanter will then be situated above Nelaton's line.

Bryant's triangle is drawn as follows. The patient lies supine and a line is drawn from the anterior superior iliac spine down towards the bed. A second line is then drawn from the anterior superior iliac spine to the tip of the greater trochanter. The third side of the triangle is a horizontal line, drawn proximally from the greater trochanter in the line of the femur to meet the first line drawn. This third line shows the amount of upward or downward displacement of the hip compared to the normal side.

It should be remembered that shortening in the femur may occasionally be *both* above and below the greater trochanter.

Telescoping of the hip, which indicates that the hip is dislocated, is assessed by pushing backwards on the lower femur with the hip and the knee flexed to a right angle and feeling the trochanter ride back on to the ilium. It is also reassessed with the leg adducted and the hip flexed. The test should then be repeated by pushing proximally

Leg Shortening

Nelaton's line

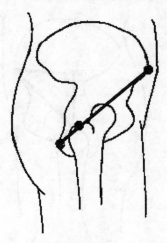

Normal

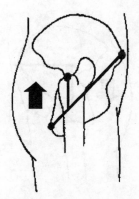

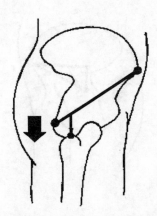

Superior displacement   **Inferior displacement**

Leg Shortening

Bryant's triangle

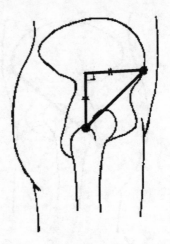

Normal

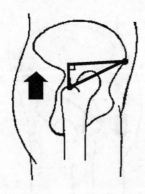

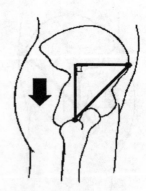

Superior displacement   **Inferior displacement**

Leg Shortening

Telescoping in flexion

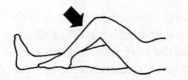 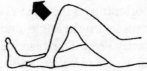

Telescoping in extension

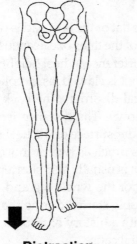 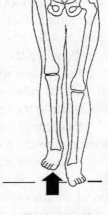

Distraction   **Compression**

---

on the foot with the hip and knee extended. The degree of telescoping is assessed by measuring the distance between the heels on both sides when the hip is pushed upwards as far as possible. This is compared with the normal position, and also with the degree of shortening when traction is exerted on the leg.

Shortening of the tibia

Shortening of the tibia can be assessed by flexing both knees to a right angle, and placing both medial malleoli exactly level. The distance at the knee between the anterior aspect of both thighs is then measured in the coronal plane. Alternatively, the distance between the top of the medial plateau of each tibia can be measured.

Shortening of the foot

The whole foot may be wasted or smaller than the opposite side, with the heel pad smaller than normal. Shortening in both the length and width of the forefoot and toes may also be seen.

In cases where the foot is flat or the heel pad is wasted, as may occur after fracture of the talus or calcaneus, there may be quite an obvious difference in heel height.

Conversely, when the foot is clawed, as in poliomyelitis or in other neurological disorders, the back of the calcaneus may be tilted down. The distance from the medial malleolus to the under surface of the heel is then increased, sometimes by as much as two or more centimetres. Despite this the foot is usually also shortened. In patients where shortening of the whole leg and foot is present the condition probably started during the growing period of childhood with a history of trauma, infection, paralysis or a congenital cause.

Leg Shortening

Shortening of the tibia

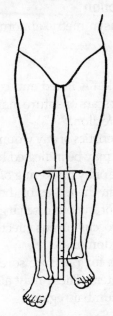

Shortening of the foot

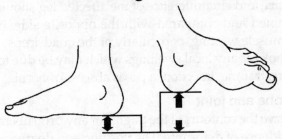

Short right heel	Long left heel
pes planus	pes cavus

Hip and Femoral Examination

Look

1. General inspection

Look for obvious asymmetry, abnormal posture or deformity.

2. Skin

The colour of the skin is noted and compared with the other side. Look for scars or suture marks indicating previous surgery or infection.

Note the characteristics of any wounds or sinuses. The direction of a sinus may be indicated by swelling above, below or to one side or by puckering of the skin. Look for granulation tissue in the edges of the sinus and at the amount and colour of any pus discharge. Yellow pus may indicate a staphylococcus aureus infection and green pus, infection with pseudomonas.

Examine the hip for pressure sores or redness over the greater trochanters. These may also occur over the lower sacrum and lumbar region.

3. Soft tissue

The size and circumference of the affected leg should be examined and compared with the opposite side. Note any muscle wasting, particularly of the quadriceps.

Look for any local swellings which may be due to tumours, trauma, infection, a psoas abscess or hernia.

4. Bone and joint

Observe the contours of the thighs for any protruberance or evidence of deformity. The position and degree of rotation of the leg, may indicate the type of dislocation or the site of a fracture.

Hip and Femoral Examination

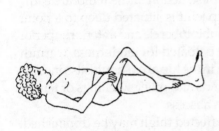

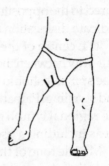

Muscle wasting　　**Asymmetrical skin folds**

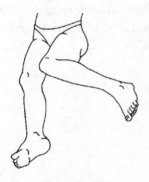

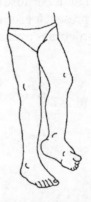

Posterior dislocation: hip flexed, adducted, internally rotated and shortened

Anterior dislocation: hip slightly flexed, abducted and externally rotated

Feel

Palpation of the hip should include palpation of the greater trochanter on each side. Its position in relationship to the anterior superior iliac spine should be compared to the opposite side, as displacement upwards may indicate dislocation or destruction of the femoral head.

The centre of the hip joint is situated deep to a point half-way between the pubic tubercle and anterior superior iliac spine. It should be palpated for tenderness, warmth and swelling. Palpation in the hip area should also include the regional lymph glands and other swellings or tender areas including a psoas abscess.

Muscle tone of the affected thigh may be diminished, as well as the muscle bulk. With the patient in the prone position gluteal tone and tenderness should be assessed including tenderness in the line of the sciatic nerve. In addition, the lumbar spine should be palpated for tender areas. This is because degenerative hip conditions, especially if present for some time, often cause a low back strain and sometimes even a prolapsed disc with sciatic irritation.

Hip and Femoral Examination

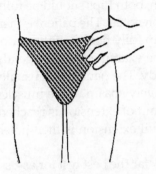

Temperature and tenderness

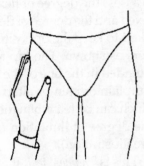

Greater trochanter

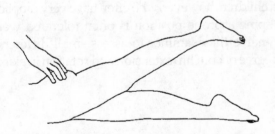

Assessment of gluteal tone

Move

1. Flexion and extension
2. Internal and external rotation
3. Abduction and adduction

Flexion and extension

To assess the degree of flexion, both hips should be fully flexed and the degree of flexion noted. The patient is then asked to keep the opposite hip fully flexed on the abdomen, as shown. The hip to be examined is then gently extended in the line of the body. The patient will usually complain of pain or alternatively spasm of the muscles which can be felt when the limit of extension is reached. The degree of limitation of full extension is then noted (see illustration).

This is *Thomas' test*. It is by far the best test for assessing any limitation of extension in the *adult*. In addition adults with a fixed flexion deformity of one or both hips will find lying face downwards on a hard examination couch extremely uncomfortable and is usually quite unnecessary in assessing limitation of extension.

In children, however, who often have very mobile hips and spine a prone position is often tolerated well and will enable the examiner to assess small differences in the degree of both hip extension and rotation in extension.

Hip and Femoral Examination

Flexion and extension

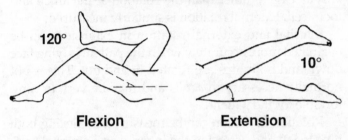

120°

Flexion

10°

Extension

Thomas' test for fixed flexion deformity
(limitation of extension)

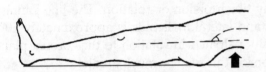

Fixed flexion deformity disguised by lumbar lordosis

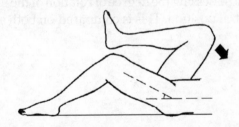

Fixed flexion deformity of left leg revealed with right hip fully flexed to eliminate lordosis

---

Internal and external rotation

Internal rotation in extension is assessed by feeling for the lateral and medial borders of each patella. The leg is then internally rotated and the *coronal* plane of the patella is assessed, rather than the rotation at the ankle and foot itself. External rotation is similarly measured.

Internal and external rotation in extension can be evaluated more accurately when the patient is lying face down and both hips are rotated in and out. This is not normally necessary in *adults* and may be very uncomfortable for the patient.

Rotation in flexion can be measured by flexing both hips to 90° and assessing the internal and external rotation.

Any rotation deformity of the tibia or femur is evaluated by palpating the medial and lateral malleoli and assessing them in relation to the patella. This will indicate any tibial torsion or rotation. The line joining the medial and lateral malleolus is approximately 20°–30° externally palpated in rotation to the coronal plane. In tibial torsion this may be much greater.

Rotation of the tibia in flexion is measured by flexing the knees to 90° and rotating the feet externally and internally and assessing the degree of rotation of the tibia from the neutral position. This is compared on both sides.

Hip and Femoral Examination

Rotation in extension

External   **Internal**

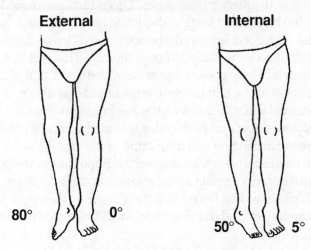

80°   0°   50°   5°

Rotation in flexion

External   **Internal**

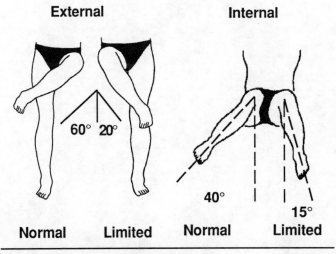

60° 20°   40°   15°

Normal   **Limited**   **Normal**   **Limited**

Abduction and adduction

Abduction and adduction of both the hips are assessed similarly. The amount of adduction from neutral is assessed in relation to the pelvis and the horizontal line joining both anterior iliac spines. This is then performed with the hips flexed to 90°. Abduction may be difficult to assess. The good leg should be abducted as far as it will go and allowed to hang out over the bed. This will lock the pelvis. The opposite leg is then abducted and the amount of abduction in relation to neutral is assessed. It is essential again to check on the line joining both anterior superior iliac spines in order to assess accurately the degree of abduction and adduction of the hips.

In children and in adults, when it is important to assess a small degree of limitation of abduction and adduction, the hips should be flexed to a right angle as shown and an assessment of abduction and adduction carried out as well.

Hip and Femoral Examination

Abduction

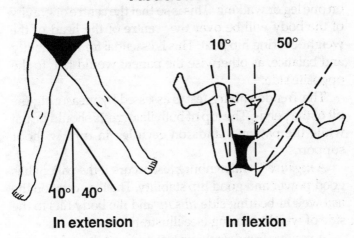

10° 50°

10° 40°

In extension **In flexion**

Adduction

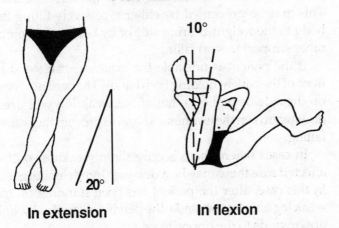

10°

20°

In extension **In flexion**

Trendelenburg test

The Trendelenburg test is a test of hip stability. It is dependent on the fact that normally the pelvis tilts upwards *away* from the side of the weight-bearing leg on standing on one leg or walking. This is so that the centre of gravity of the body will be over the centre of the head of the weight-bearing hip joint. This is essential for hip stability and balance, as otherwise the patient would fall to the opposite side.

The Trendelenburg test is assessed by measuring the tilt of the pelvis. The top of both iliac crests should be felt while the patient stands on each leg in turn without support.

A *negative* Trendelenburg test occurs if the patient has good power and good hip stability. The iliac crest on the *non* weight-bearing side *tilts up* and the body tilts to the side of weight-bearing (see illustration).

A *positive* Trendelenburg test occurs if the pelvis sags *downwards* to the *opposite* side on weight-bearing. The patient will also then tend to fall to the opposite side. This may be prevented by either excessively tilting the body to the weight-bearing side or by holding a chair or other support to stop falling.

If the patient is unstable the examiner can stand in front of the patient holding both hands. The patient's hand on the side opposite to that of the weak hip will press downwards on the examiner's hand to prevent the patient falling.

In cases where there is only slight weakness on the affected side there may be a delayed Trendelenburg test. In this case, after the patient has been standing on the weak leg for a few seconds, the pelvis will gradually sink downwards to the opposite side.

A Simple Guide to Orthopaedics

Trendelenburg Test

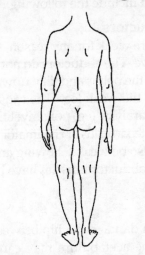

Negative Trendelenburg test — normal	Positive Trendelenburg test — abnormal

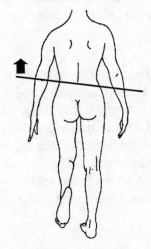 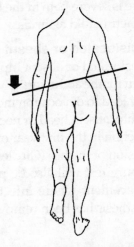

Pelvis tilts upwards	Pelvis sags downwards on unaffected side

The common causes of a positive Trendelenburg test are illustrated and include the following:

1. Weak hip abductors

If the abductors are weak for any reason, the Trendelenburg test is positive. The abductors do not have enough power to support the pelvis and tilt it upwards when the patient stands on the weak leg. The cause of weak abductors may be paralysis (eg. poliomyelitis), or wasting and pain due to osteoarthritis or rheumatoid arthritis. The abductors may also be weak following an operation on the hip when the abductor muscles have been detached or damaged.

2. Damaged hip

Conditions which damage the hip between the greater trochanter and the acetabulum may cause instability. These include fractures of the neck or head of the femur or damage to the acetabulum. Instability also occurs if there is severe pain in the hip secondary to osteoarthritis or rheumatoid arthritis.

3. Dislocated or absent hip

A dislocated or absent hip will mean that there is no fulcrum for the abductors to work across. Conditions which may lead to dislocation include congenital dislocation of the hip, absent head or neck of the femur due to previous infection in the first year of life (Tom Smith's disease), or excision of the hip (Girdlestone procedure). The Trendelenburg test will also be positive after a failed total hip replacement where infection has supervened and the prosthesis has been removed.

Positive Trendelenburg Test
Common Causes

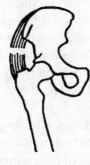

Weak hip abductors

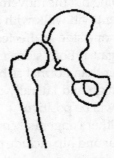

Dislocated hip

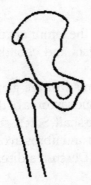

Absent hip joint

Hip and Femoral Conditions

Congenital abnormalities

In the older child and adult, examination of an untreated congenital dislocation usually reveals a short leg with limitation of abduction in flexion. There may be telescoping but the movements will usually be painless. The patient will walk with an unstable and short leg gait, if only one side is affected, and will waddle with a swaying gait if both sides are affected. The pelvis will look wider than normal as both hips and trochanters are riding high and laterally on the ilium. The Trendelenburg test will be positive.

Other congenital conditions sometimes affecting the femur and hip include phocomelia due to drugs, such as thalidomide, used in the first trimester of pregnancy, as well as genetic causes. Coxa valga or vara, fibrous dysplasia, diaphyseal aclasis and other genetic anomalies may also occur and are discussed later.

Neoplasia

Primary neoplasms of the femur are uncommon and include benign bone cysts and chondroblastoma of the femoral head.

Malignant neoplasms include giant cell tumours of the epiphysis, osteogenic sarcoma of the metaphysis and Ewing's sarcoma of the shaft. Soft tissue neoplasms such as rhabdomyosarcoma and fibrosarcoma are rare. Multiple painful lipomata (Dercum's disease) may occur in obese people.

Hip and Femoral Conditions

Congenital abnormalities

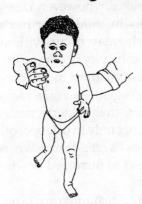

Phocomelia

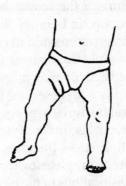

Asymmetrical skin folds eg. CDH

Neoplasia

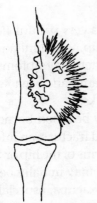

X-ray appearance of osteogenic sarcoma of femoral metaphysis

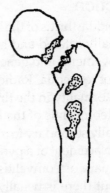

X-ray appearance of secondary tumour deposits with fractured neck of femur

Trauma

Fractures of the hip and femur are common and are usually easily differentiated from other hip conditions by a history and examination. Occasionally, however, a stress fracture of the femur, especially in children or in the osteoporotic bone of the elderly, may occur without obvious trauma and may cause difficulty in diagnosis.

In children, a stress fracture secondary to unaccustomed activity may mimic an osteogenic sarcoma radiologically with new bone formation. In the elderly, pathological fractures may also occur, not only in osteoporotic bone, but also in conditions such as Paget's disease where multiple stress fractures may lead to increased bowing before a complete fracture occurs.

Dislocations of the hip due to acute trauma are usually easy to diagnose. Occasionally there may be difficulty if associated with previous paralysis or congenital anomalies.

Infection

Pyogenic arthritis of the hip causes a very painful, flexed, externally rotated and adducted hip, with limitation of all movements and generalised systemic symptoms and signs of toxaemia. Radiological examination may show no abnormality in the first 2–3 weeks.

Osteomyelitis of the femur may be blood-borne, but is usually secondary to a compound fracture, an infected hip replacement or a pyogenic arthritis of the hip or knee. In primary osteomyelitis the X-ray may initially be normal, but there is usually severe toxaemia, especially in children.

Hip and Femoral Conditions

Trauma

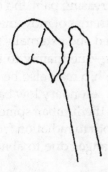

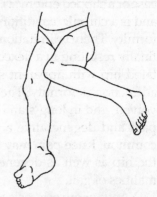

X-ray appearance of a trochanteric fracture

Posterior dislocation of the hip

Infection

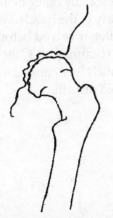

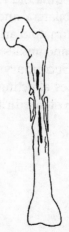

X-ray appearance of pyogenic arthritis

X-ray appearance of osteomyelitis

Arthritis

Osteoarthritis of the hip is common and may be primary (unknown cause) or secondary to previous fracture, dislocation or other hip abnormalities such as Perthes' disease or a slipped epiphysis. Osteoarthritis has a slow onset and is a chronic condition with increasing pain and deformity. There is limitation at the extremes of movement, finally resulting in a flexed, adducted and externally rotated hip with apparent shortening, due mainly to the adduction deformity. The opposite hip may also be involved, and in long-standing cases, secondary low back pain and degenerative arthritis of the lumbar spine is common. Knee pain may be due both to radiation from the hip as well as degenerative changes due to abnormalities of gait.

X-rays show sclerosis and cyst formation, with diminution of the joint space and osteophyte formation of the femoral head and acetabulum.

Rheumatoid arthritis may also involve the hip. It is often bilateral and acute. There is usually other evidence of rheumatoid arthritis, particularly of the hands, wrists, knees and ankles and these are often involved before the hips. Secondary osteoarthritis is common. Other arthritides affecting the hip are much less common than either osteoarthritis or rheumatoid arthritis.

Hip and Femoral Conditions

Arthritis

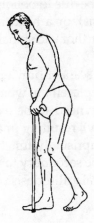

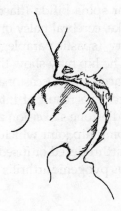

Patient with osteoarthritis

X-ray appearance of an osteoarthritic hip with cysts and sclerosis

Miscellaneous conditions

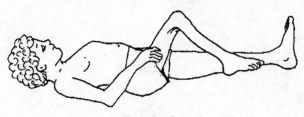

Paralysis

Miscellaneous conditions

Other conditions involving the hip and femur include Paget's disease, where the femur is thickened and bowed, and this may occasionally cause a pathological fracture. Paralysis of the hip and thigh may be due to poliomyelitis or spina bifida (flaccid paralysis), or a head injury, stroke, cerebral palsy or cervical or thoracic spinal cord injury (spastic paraplegia).

The hip may show the surgical scars of previous hip replacements. Occasionally, a hip replacement which has failed as a result of infection may need to be excised (Girdlestone's excision arthroplasty), resulting in a telescoping hip joint which may be suprisingly functional. An arthrodesed or fused hip may be secondary to a previous pyogenic arthritis or a surgical arthrodesis.

Knee and Tibial Examination

Look

1. General inspection
Compare both knees looking for obvious asymmetry or deformity.

2. Skin
Inspect the colour of the skin of the knee, thigh and leg and compare with the opposite side and also look for wounds, scars or sinuses on the front, sides and back.

3. Soft tissue
Look for swellings over all aspects of the knee. Swelling above the front of the knee may be an enlarged supra-patellar bursa (an outpouching of the knee joint itself). Below the knee there may be an enlarged infra- patellar bursa (clergyman's knee), and on the front of the patella an enlarged prepatellar bursa (house maid's knee).

Swelling in the popliteal fossa may be a Baker's cyst or a popliteal aneurysm. Calf swelling may be due to a ruptured Baker's cyst or a deep vein thrombosis.

If the knee is not obviously swollen, look for filling out of the gutters on either side of the patella and this may be made more obvious by 'milking' down synovial fluid from just above the knee. It may indicate a joint effusion or synovial thickening.

Check for wasting of the quadriceps and calf muscles.

4. Bone and joint
Look at the knee alignment, noting the presence of genu recurvatum, genu valgum or genu varum or flexion deformity. Look at the position of the patella. Look for bony swellings including tumours, possible fractures and infection.

Knee and Tibial Examination

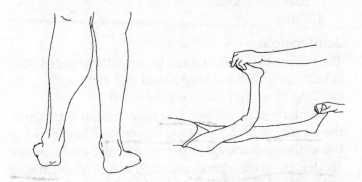

Ruptured Baker's cyst　　　　**Genu recurvatum**

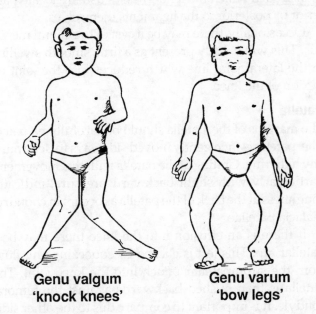

Genu valgum　　　　　　　　**Genu varum**
'knock knees'　　　　　　　　**'bow legs'**

Feel

1. Joint margin
2. Patella
3. Back of the knee
4. Other

Joint margin

The margin of the joint should be carefully palpated. This is best done with the knee flexed to a right angle. Any swelling or tenderness should be noted.

Tenderness in the joint line may indicate damage of the menisci or of the collateral ligaments. The exact location of the tenderness is important in making a diagnosis. Tenderness of the ligaments usually occurs on the medial or lateral side of the joint, quite distinct from injury of a meniscus in which the tenderness is usually located anterior or posterior to the ligaments themselves.

Occasionally, there may be a cyst of the lateral meniscus. This will usually present as a firm, smooth swelling in the lateral joint line which reduces into the joint on flexion of the knee.

Patella

The margins of the patella should be carefully palpated. The patella is then gently moved sideways to determine any tethering. Grating of the patella with this movement, particularly with slight backward pressure, indicates roughness at the back of the patella as occurs in chondromalacia patellae.

If there is an effusion into the knee there may be a patellar tap. This test is elicited by squeezing any fluid from the suprapatellar pouch into the knee joint. The patella is then pushed backwards against the femoral condyle. It is important to compare this to the other side.

Knee and Tibial Examination

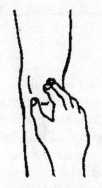

Temperature, tenderness, swellings

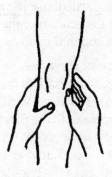

Joint margins

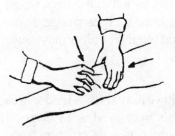

Patellar tap testing for knee effusion

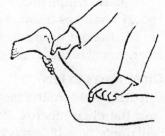

Palpate popliteal fossa for cyst, aneurysm, lymph nodes

If there is too much or too little fluid a patellar tap cannot be elicited. A tap may sometimes be detected with a small amount of fluid by pushing the patella sideways.

The patella should also be gently pushed from side to side, particularly laterally. This may elicit pain in recurrent dislocation of the patella. The opposite side should be compared in all cases.

Back of the knee

Palpate the back of the knee for tenderness and swelling. This is best done with the knee flexed to about 60° and if possible with the patient lying prone. In osteoarthritis an outpouching of the synovium may occur, called a Baker's cyst. A popliteal aneurysm may produce a pulsatile swelling in the back of the knee over which a bruit may be heard. If an aneurysm is suspected the peripheral vessels should be palpated, particularly the posterior tibial artery behind the medial malleolus, and the dorsalis pedis artery pulse between the first and second metatarsal bones. It is important to compare the pulsation in both limbs.

Popliteal lymph nodes may be felt at the back of the knee. Conditions below the knee such as pyogenic arthritis, a tumour, or an infected wound or ulcer may cause enlargement of these nodes.

Other areas to feel

Palpation of the front of the knee may show a tender area over the tibial tubercle. This may be due to Osgood Schlatter's type of osteochondritis — a traction apophysitis, often occurring in adolescent boys. Tenderness above the tibial tubercle may be due to partial or complete rupture of the ligamentum patellae. Tenderness over the patella itself may indicate a fracture or other injury, or a prepatellar bursa. Swelling above the patella sometimes signifies damage to the muscles above the patella or an effusion into the knee joint due to arthritis or infection.

Swelling of the knee itself is usually due to fluid, synovium, bone or a combination of these. Various types of fluid produce knee swellings. These include: synovial fluid which may follow cartilage injury, blood secondary to ligamentous damage or a fracture, and pus resulting from infection.

Synovial thickening may be due to acute or chronic synovitis or rarely a synoviosarcoma. Rheumatoid arthritis, osteoarthritis and many other arthritides may cause both synovial thickening and an effusion.

Move

1. Collateral ligaments and menisci
2. Cruciate ligaments
3. Flexion and extension

Collateral ligaments and menisci

The collateral ligaments should be examined carefully. This is best done with the knee in about 20° or 30° of flexion as the cruciates and the posterior capsule lock the knee when it is fully extended. It is important, as always, to compare both sides. Rupture of the collateral ligaments may often be associated with meniscal damage and tears.

Examination of the medial and lateral menisci involves rotating the knee into valgus and varus positions, and flexing and extending the joint. The finger tips placed on the medial or lateral joint lines respectively may feel a catching or clicking of a loose piece of meniscus. A loose piece of bone is sometimes detached, such as an osteochondral fragment from a fracture or from an osteochondritis dissecans. These may be felt in any part of the knee.

McMurray's test

This test is used to assist in the diagnosis of suspected meniscal tears, excluding bucket handle tears. The knee should be flexed to 90°, the examiner then externally or internally rotates the foot, and slowly extends the knee joint, with the leg held in rotation. External rotation is used to test for lesions of the medial meniscus, and internal rotation for lateral meniscal tears. A normal knee will often 'click' when rotated in flexion. This can be differentiated from a positive McMurray's test, however, where the torn meniscus will produce a click that is louder, and often palpable. In addition, a positive McMurray's test will often produce pain.

Knee and Tibial Examination

Collateral ligaments

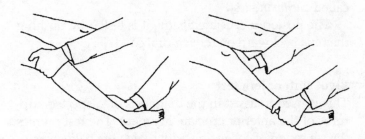

**Testing medial
collateral ligament—
knee flexed at 20°**

**Testing lateral
collateral ligament—
knee flexed at 20°**

Menisci

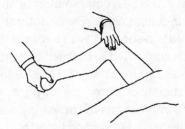

**McMurray's test — internal and external rotation
of the leg, both in abduction and adduction**

Cruciate ligaments

An anterior cruciate ligament is tested for laxity by pulling the upper tibia forward on the femoral condyles with the knee flexed to a right angle. It can also be assessed by feeling for anterior laxity with the muscles relaxed, the heel on the bed and the knee flexed to about 20°. This is called *Lachman's test*.

The posterior cruciate ligament is tested by pushing the tibia backward on the femoral condyle.

Pivot shift or jerk test

This is used to assist in the diagnosis of suspected ruptures of the anterior cruciate ligament. The test mimics the sensation of collapsing with which the patients may present. The technique involves pushing the head of the tibia anteriorly, while the lower limb is internally rotated, and a valgus force is applied. While in this position, the knee should be extended and flexed, which will alternately sublux, and reduce the lateral tibial plateau on the femoral condyle. Tibial reduction may occur with a sharp, visible, or palpable jerk at about 30° of flexion.

There may also be a combination of anterior cruciate and medial ligament rupture with anteromedial instability. This is often associated with a tear of the medial meniscus which is attached to the medial ligament. Rupture of the lateral ligament sometimes also occurs with posterior cruciate rupture, resulting in posterolateral instability. Combinations of these may also occur. More specialised tests are performed by orthopaedic surgeons to evaluate the exact degree of ligamentous damage in the knee joint, but the final diagnosis is usually made at arthroscopy.

Knee and Tibial Examination

Cruciate ligaments

anterior

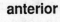

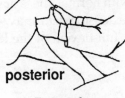

posterior

Draw sign

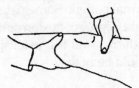

Lachman's test

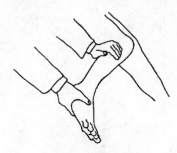

Pivot shift test

Extension

40°

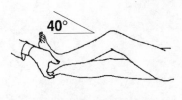

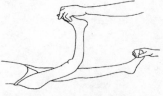

**Limited extension —
fixed flexion deformity**

**Hyperextension —
genu recurvatum**

Flexion and extension

The knee should be examined carefully for movement and the degree of flexion and extension noted. If there is any limitation, this should be compared with the opposite side because there are often slight variations in the normal patient. Some patients with normal knees have a slight degree of flexion or hyperextension deformity. Any tenderness on full extension or full flexion of the knee should be noted.

Knee and Tibial Conditions

Congenital abnormalities

Congenital conditions which may affect the knee and tibia include limb deficiencies such as phocomelia and over-growth such as macrodactyly and congenital lymphangiectasis. Congenital contractures of the knee may occur with webbing and arthrogryposis (generalised collagen replacement of muscles and associated with contractures). Genu recurvatum may be due to congenital shortening of the quadriceps or more commonly it is associated with maternal oestrogen excess prior to birth, together with an intrauterine malposition of the foetus in the last few weeks of pregnancy.

Genu valgum or varum are common and when severe are due to growth imbalance at the upper tibial or lower femoral growth epiphyses.

Neoplasia

Primary neoplasms of the tibia may be benign or malignant. Unlike the femur, however, secondary neoplasms are uncommon. Benign neoplasms include osteochondroma and non-ossifying fibroma. Malignant neoplasms include giant cell tumours in the epiphysis, osteogenic sarcoma of the metaphysis and Ewing's sarcoma of the diaphysis.

Trauma

Osteochondritis dissecans usually occurs on the lateral side of the medial femoral condyle. There is damage of the cartilage and underlying bone with death of a small part of the condyle. This may revascularise or die completely and be detached into the knee joint as a loose osteocartilaginous body.

Knee and Tibial Conditions

Congenital abnormalities

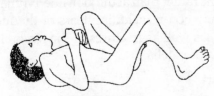

Webbed knee

Neoplasia

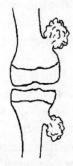

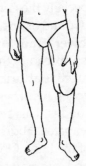

X-ray appearance of an osteochondroma

Osteogenic sarcoma

Trauma

Meniscal injuries

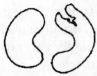

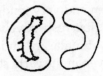

Tear of anterior or posterior poles

Bucket-handle tear

With the knee flexed to a 90° angle there is usually localised tenderness just above the joint margin on the lateral side of the medial femoral condyle. Occasionally the detachment may be situated elsewhere. It is above the joint line rather than at the joint line. Numerous other injuries may occur, including tears of the menisci and ligaments, as well as fractures of the femoral condyles, upper tibia or patella.

Infection

Infection may involve the knee joint. This is usually acute, and may be due to a blood-borne infection from a primary focus elsewhere, such as the throat or genitourinary tract and especially the gonococcus. It may also follow a penetrating wound or an operation on the knee. Osteomyelitis of the lower femur, or less commonly of the upper tibia, may also spread to the knee joint.

In infective arthritis of the knee, the joint is hot, tender and swollen, with systemic upset and enlarged inguinal lymph nodes. This swelling extends above the knee into the suprapatellar bursa, which is continuous with the joint space of the knee. Occasionally the infection can be low-grade and this may occur following early antibiotic therapy, or with an organism causing chronic infection such as the tubercle bacillus.

Infection of the prepatellar or infrapatellar bursae is usually due to direct local infection. The bursae are red, swollen and very tender over the front of the patella or upper tibia respectively, and the regional inguinal lymph nodes are enlarged and tender. The underlying knee joint however, in the early stages, is unaffected.

Knee and Tibial Conditions
Infection

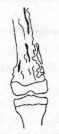

X-ray appearance
of osteomyelitis

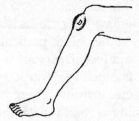

Infrapatellar bursitis

Arthritis

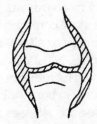

Rheumatoid arthritis

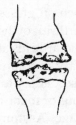

X-ray appearance of
osteoarthritis

Miscellaneous conditions

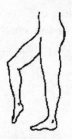

Paralytic leg

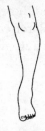

Paget's disease of the tibia

Arthritis

Apart from an infective arthritis, the two common arthritides affecting the knee joint are rheumatoid and osteoarthritis.

Rheumatoid arthritis is often bilateral and usually involves other joints, particularly of the hands, wrists, ankles and feet. The onset is usually fairly acute, but the joint is much less warm, swollen and tender than in a pyogenic arthritis. There is often considerable synovial swelling as well, and it is this, in the subacute and chronic stages, that is often more obvious than the actual effusion itself. Radiological examination in the earlier stages merely shows osteoporosis of the lower femur and upper tibia. In the later stages there is diminution of the joint space which progresses to secondary osteoarthritis.

Osteoarthritis of the knee is much more common than rheumatoid arthritis and may be primary or alternatively secondary to trauma or other causes. Most cases are probably secondary to trauma. This will include not only ligamentous or meniscal damage, but also bony or cartilage damage. Asymmetrical joint surface stresses may occur in genu varum or valgum and also with irregular joint surfaces following a fracture of the upper tibia, lower femur or patella. X-rays in osteoarthritis usually show diminution of joint space with osteophyte formation and sclerosis and there may also be evidence of an aetiological factor. Rarer causes of arthritis of the knee joint include other autoimmune diseases and psoriasis.

Miscellaneous conditions

Another condition affecting the knee and tibia is Paget's disease which causes thickening and bowing of the tibiae. Causes of paralysis of the muscles around and below the knee include spinal cord or sciatic nerve injury, spina bifida and poliomyelitis.

Ankle and Foot Examination

Look

1. General inspection

Inspect the ankle and foot, comparing with the opposite foot. Note any obvious asymmetry or deformity.

2. Skin

Look for sores, scars or colour change. Sores or ulcers may be associated with poor circulation or with an injury or infection.

Callosities on the toes, on the sides or plantar surface of the foot may be due to an underlying structural abnormality or to badly fitting footwear.

Examine the nails for clubbing or deformity.

3. Soft tissues

Look for any swelling, noting possible causes such as gouty tophi over the first metatarso-phalangeal joint, rheumatoid nodules over the achilles tendon, swellings resulting from trauma, infection or ganglia.

Look for muscle contractures as a cause of deformity such as in Dupuytren's contracture, Volkmann's ischaemic contracture or paralysis.

4. Bone and joint

The deformities of the foot should be divided into those of the hindfoot, forefoot and toes. Look posteriorly for valgus or varus deformity of the heels and then anteriorly for forefoot deformity. The forefoot may show clawing (pes cavus) or flattening (pes planus). Look at the toes for the presence of clawing or hallux valgus. Look for changes of rheumatoid or osteoarthritis and note any bony swellings such as exostoses.

Ankle and Foot Examination

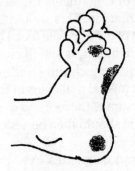

Callosities

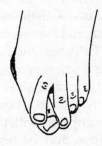

Hallux valgus

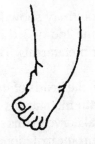

Varus deformity

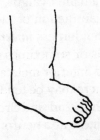

Valgus deformity

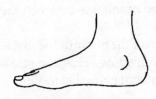

Pes planus

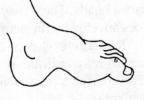

Pes cavus

Feel

The examiner should feel the foot with the back of the proximal phalanx of the middle or ring fingers to assess the warmth of the toes, foot and ankle. This should be compared with the identical part of the opposite foot. The foot should then be palpated for tenderness and fluctuation. Palpation should be systematic, including feeling for tenderness over the lateral or medial malleolus of the ankle in injuries and over the dorsum of the foot and over the 5th metatarsal head. Sensation should then be tested and compared with the opposite side.

There may be tenderness and callosities over the proximal interphalangeal joints of the toes (corns), or over the 1st metatarso-phalangeal joint (bunion), associated with a hallux valgus.

Examination of the sole of the foot may show localised tenderness *under* the heads of the 2nd or 3rd metatarsals or sometimes over the other metatarsals. This is called anterior metatarsalgia.

There may be tenderness *between* the heads of the 1st and 2nd, 2nd and 3rd, or 3rd and 4th metatarsals. This may indicate a neuroma of the digital nerve in this space which has developed secondary to chronic irritation. This pain is made worse by squeezing the forefoot between the 1st and the 5th metatarsals which compresses the enlarged and inflamed nerve situated between the metatarsal heads. There may also be numbness between the toes affected by the neuroma.

Tenderness over the dorsum of the necks of the metatarsals may indicate a 'march' fracture. This is a stress fracture due to excessive or unaccustomed standing or walking.

Ankle and Foot Examination

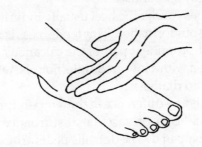

Temperature

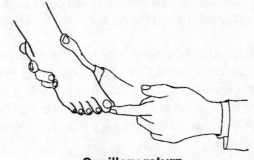

Capillary return

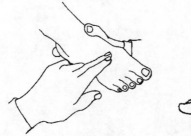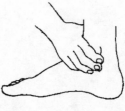

Dorsalis pedis artery   **Posterior tibial artery**

There may be tenderness under the longitudinal arch. This is usually the result of foot strain, especially in heavy patients with poor muscles.

Tenderness under the heel usually indicates a plantar fasciitis or spur formation. This tenderness is just anterior to the most prominent part of the calcaneus. It may also be associated with a low grade infection elsewhere or with a rheumatoid diathesis.

If there is any difference in the temperature of the feet or any likelihood of vascular disturbance the pulses should be palpated. The dorsalis pedis artery is situated between the proximal part of the 1st and 2nd metatarsal shafts. The posterior tibial artery is situated half way between the medial malleolus and the point of the heel. The capillary return and the colour of the toes should be noted.

The left and right sides should be carefully compared and any difference noted. The actual distribution of tender areas on the underside of the foot is illustrated.

There may be sensory impairment and this is illustrated later and will help localise the level of neurological impairment.

Ankle and Foot Tenderness

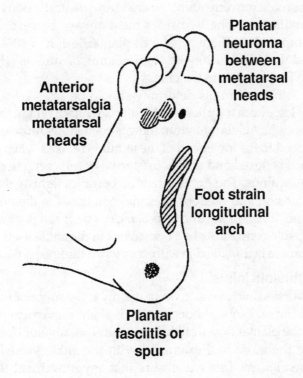

Plantar neuroma between metatarsal heads

Anterior metatarsalgia metatarsal heads

Foot strain longitudinal arch

Plantar fasciitis or spur

Move

Movements of the ankle and foot are divided into:
1. Movements of the ankle
2. Movements of the subtaloid and midtarsal joints
3. Movements of the forefoot and toes

Ankle

The main movements of the ankle are plantarflexion and dorsiflexion. The two sides must always be carefully compared. In the normal foot plantarflexion is 40°–50° and dorsiflexion 20°–30° from neutral. Neutral is when the foot is at 90° to the tibia.

A fixed equinus deformity should be assessed with the knee both fully flexed and fully extended. Where there is a tight Achilles tendon, the gastrocnemius muscle attached to the lower end of the femur is relaxed when the knee is flexed and allows for partial or full correction of the equinus. The Achilles tendon becomes tight again in extension and the foot goes into equinus. On the other hand, if equinus is due to local factors such as a posterior capsule contracture or a bony block in the ankle itself, no increase in dorsiflexion will occur when the knee is flexed.

Subtaloid joints

Inversion and eversion occur mainly at the subtaloid and midtarsal joints, although there is slight movement also in the plantar flexed ankle joint itself. The subtaloid joints are therefore best examined with the ankle locked in dorsiflexion. This will ensure that any movement then occurring is at the subtaloid or midtarsal joints or even further forward in the forefoot itself, rather than in the ankle.

About 60° of inversion and 30°– 40° of eversion of the foot is usually possible at the midtarsal joints. In condi-

Ankle and Foot Examination

Plantarflexion and dorsiflexion

Fixed equinus deformity of right foot

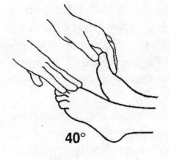

40°

Plantarflexion

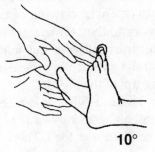

10°

Dorsiflexion

Inversion and eversion

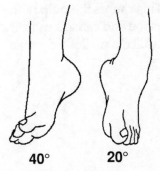

40° **20°**

Inversion

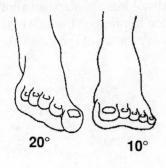

20° **10°**

Eversion

tions affecting the subtaloid or midtarsal joints, such as infection, this movement may be limited or absent.

Forefoot and toes

The third set of movements involves the forefoot and toes. Further inversion and eversion may be present in the forefoot. In addition, a small degree of adduction or abduction is possible.

Deformities such as hallux valgus, with limitation of movement or clawing of the toes, may also be present. Injury to the 1st metatarso-phalangeal joint can also result in stiffness of this joint ('hallux rigidus'). In some paralytic conditions there may also be clawing or 'cocking up' of the big toe.

The 2nd–5th toes can be 'clawed' at the proximal interphalangeal joints due to poor intrinsic muscles of the foot ('hammer toe'). There is often a callosity or painful 'corn' over the dorsum of this joint due to pressure of shoes over this joint. In addition the proximal phalanx is usually dorsally dislocated or subluxed at the metatarso-phalangeal joint.

Occasionally the flexion deformity is mainly at the distal inter-phalangeal joint. This causes the pulp of the toe to press on the sole of the shoe and cause a callosity over the tip of the toe. This is called a mallet toe.

Ankle and Foot Conditions

Congenital abnormalities

Congenital conditions can be divided into limb deficiency, such as phocomelia, and limb overgrowth such as macrodactyly.

In congenital lymphangioma or similar conditions the whole limb may be enlarged, and sometimes the whole side of the body. The individual digits may be fused, and this is referred to as syndactyly, or individual joints may be stiff due to conditions such as arthrogryposis.

Talipes equino varus is usually due to a congenital deformity in which the foot is inverted (varus), and plantarflexed (equinus). The opposite to this is talipes calcaneo valgus where the foot is dorsiflexed and everted. In true talipes equino varus or calcaneo valgus, sensation and power are initially normal. The spine, however, should always be examined in all foot deformities as there may occasionally be an associated spina bifida or myelomeningocele. In such cases there are usually also sensory disturbances, together with motor weakness.

The feet may also be deformed. There may be clawing of the toes, overriding of the little toe or a hallux valgus.

Neoplasia

Neoplasms of the ankle and foot are rare. The neoplasms may be malignant, such as a melanoma, or benign soft tissue swellings such as a ganglion. Other neoplasms include enchondroma, ecchondroma and chondrosarcoma. Exostoses may occur, usually due to rubbing of a shoe over a bony prominence such as the 1st metatarsal head, the 5th metatarsal base or the calcaneus.

Ankle and Foot Conditions

Congenital abnormalities

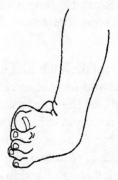

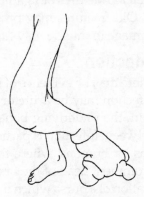

Talipes equino varus

Macrodactyly

Neoplasia

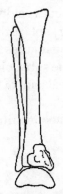

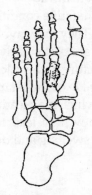

X-ray appearance of a
giant cell tumour of the
distal tibia

X-ray appearance of a
chondrosarcoma of
second metatarsal

Trauma

The different varieties of ankle and foot injuries are too numerous to be discussed here. In general, however, injuries may be classified as either acute or chronic, and then as fractures or ligamentous injuries.

Old fractures may produce deformity, and vascular damage to muscle may cause a fibrous contracture.

Infection

There may be evidence of infection of the ankle and foot. Infection may be acute or chronic and may involve the skin, the underlying bone or joint, or the soft tissue in between. Infection is particularly common in hallux valgus, or bunions, where the rubbing of a shoe over the prominent head of the first metatarsal results in the formation of a bursa which may break through the skin and become secondarily infected.

Arthritis

Osteoarthritis

Degenerative conditions are common in the elderly patient. They may involve the ankle or the joints of the foot. They are particularly common following injuries such as a fracture of the calcaneus involving the subtaloid joint, the ankle or the 1st metatarso-phalangeal joint of the big toe (which may lead to hallux rigidus).

They may lead to degenerative osteoarthritis with pain, swelling and deformity.

Ankle and Foot Conditions

Trauma

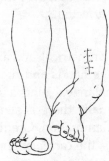

Old trauma

Infection

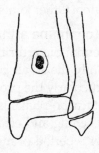

X-ray appearance of a
Brodie's abscess

Osteoarthritis

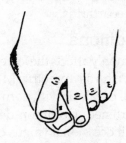

Hallux valgus: osteoarthritis
of 1st MTP joint

Metabolic arthritis

In gout, the metatarso-phalangeal joint of the big toe is often involved. Involvement may be unilateral or bilateral. After a time, the skin may break down with extrusion of a white chalky material which contains uric acid crystals. There may be other evidence of gout including gouty tophi of the fingers, hands, ears and over the olecranon. Other joints may also be affected.

Autoimmune arthritis

Rheumatoid arthritis is usually symmetrical and affects mainly the small joints of both the hands and the feet, particularly the proximal interphalangeal joints and the metacarpo-phalangeal joints. Initially there is synovial thickening and effusion with inflammation. Gradually, over a period of months or years, the cartilage and the bones of the small joints are destroyed leading to secondary osteoarthritis. In addition, the overlying tendons may be attenuated and destroyed leading to joint subluxation, especially of the metacarpo-phalangeal and proximal interphalangeal joints.

Rheumatoid arthritis in children is called Still's disease. It may leave the child with multiple deformities of the hands, feet and other joints with growth retardation and secondary osteoarthritis.

Paralytic conditions

Poliomyelitis commonly affects the lower limbs more than the upper limbs. It is an asymmetrical, flaccid, lower motor neurone type of paralysis with normal sensation. The limb is often shortened. Common deformities are an equinus ankle with occasional valgus or varus deformities, together with clawing of the foot and toes.

Ankle and Foot Conditions

Metabolic arthritis

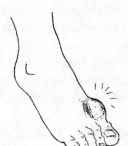

Gout

Autoimmune arthritis

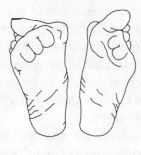

Rheumatoid feet

Paralysis

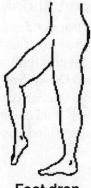

Foot drop

Damage to the *thoracic* spine usually results in *spasticity* with an *upper motor neurone* type paralysis affecting both lower limbs. Fractures of the *lumbar spine,* on the other hand, may lead to a *lower motor neurone* flaccid paralysis.

Spastic paralysis may also be due to birth trauma, stroke, or congenital anomalies. In these conditions both feet are usually held in equinus and the muscles are not wasted. The reflexes are usually increased asymmetrically. Sensation is often virtually normal.

Damage to peripheral nerves may occur in injuries such as open wounds or in dislocation of joints such as the hip and knee. Both sensory loss and flaccid paralysis may result.

Ulceration and bed sores, also known as decubitus ulcers, may occur in paralysis if there is an associated sensory loss, as the patient is unable to feel areas where there is excessive or prolonged pressure. This ulceration usually involves the point of the heels as well as the greater trochanters and the sacrum. Such sores generally do not occur in poliomyelitis patients where sensation is normal.

Miscellaneous conditions

Other conditions include tenderness over the achilles tendon and its sheath due to excessive use, thickening of the fascia under the longitudinal arch, associated with clawing of the toes, and Dupuytren's fascial contracture, often associated with a similar condition in the hands. Curved overgrowth and thickening of the toe nails, particularly of the big toe, is called onychogryphosis.

Ankle and Foot Conditions

Miscellaneous conditions

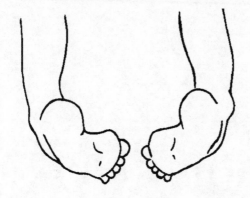

Bilateral spastic talipes equino varus

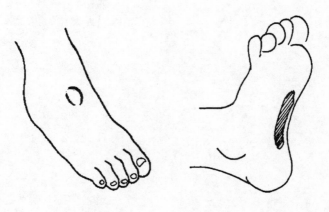

Ganglion   **Plantar fibromatosis**

Neurological Examination of the Lower Limb

Neurological assessment

1. Look
2. Feel — sensation
3. Move — tone
   power
   reflexes
   co-ordination

Peripheral nerve lesions

1. Lateral cutaneous nerve of the thigh
2. Femoral
3. Sciatic
4. Common peroneal
5. Tibial

Neurological Assessment

Lower limb neurological deficits may be the result of cerebral, spinal or peripheral nerve lesions. These causes are discussed in more detail in Chapter 11: 'Neurological and Spinal Conditions'.

The neurological examination of the lower limbs should include an assessment of tone, power, reflexes, sensation and co-ordination.

Look

The limbs should be inspected initially for wasting, deformity, contractures, and shortening. Skin changes such as discolouration, ulceration, or hair loss may also be noted and are usually due to either vascular or neurological pathology.

Posture of the limbs may give a clue as to the possible aetiology of paralysis. This may include an adduction deformity of the lower limbs ('scissoring') in a patient with a spastic diplegia, and occasionally athetoid movements or fasciculation. Shortening of any part of the limb may indicate that a neurological condition has been present since birth or childhood, for example spina bifida or poliomyelitis. The contralateral 'normal' lower limb should always be inspected for comparison.

Feel

Muscle bulk and temperature changes should be compared by palpation of both lower limbs. The bladder should be palpated for enlargement if there is any history of urinary retention or difficulty in micturating.

Dermatomes
Lower Limb

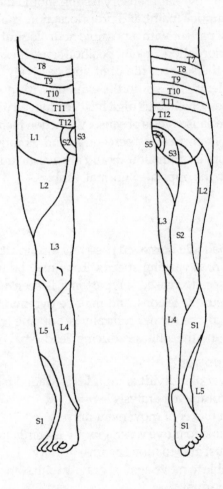

Anterior   **Posterior**

Sensation

The dermatomes of the lower limb are illustrated. It should be noted, however, that there is often considerable sensory overlap. Sensory testing should include light touch, pinprick (pain), and proprioception, as a minimum for every patient with a possible neurological lesion.

Proprioception, or joint position sense is examined by holding the sides of the digit and passively dorsi- and plantarflexing it, while the patient with eyes closed, nominates whether the digit has been moved up or down. More specialised tests of sensory function include examination of temperature perception and vibration sense.

Sensory examination should always include comparison with the opposite, 'normal' limb.

Move

Tone

The limb should be moved passively through its full range of motion, at varying speeds. Tone may be normal, increased, or decreased. Hypertonia is seen with upper motor neurone lesions, and may be pyramidal or extrapyramidal, the former typically producing 'clasp knife' rigidity, and the latter producing 'lead pipe' rigidity.

Muscle power

The power of individual muscles is graded from 0 to 5:

    0 — complete paralysis
    1 — a flicker of movement only
    2 — able to move when gravity is eliminated
    3 — just able to move against gravity
    4 — able to move against gravity with some resistance
    5 — normal

Adding '1/2' or '+' signifies a power in between two grades. The importance of assessing muscle power is

Muscle Power

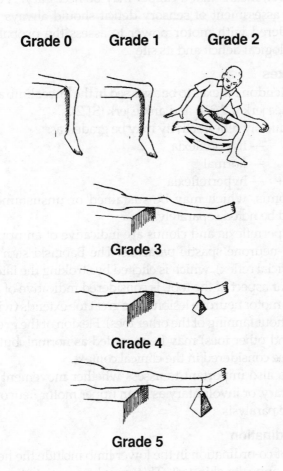

Grade 0   Grade 1   Grade 2

Grade 3

Grade 4

Grade 5

based on the fact that a power of more than 3 in the knee extensors, or in the foot dorsiflexors, will mean that a caliper will not be necessary. A power less than three, however, means that a caliper may be necessary. A detailed assessment of sensory deficit should always be considered with motor power to assess the probable neurological deficit and its site.

Reflexes

Deep tendon reflexes to be assessed in the lower limb are the knee jerk (L2,3,4) and ankle jerk (S1,2).

Clinically reflex activity may be graded as:

+ — hyporeflexia

++ — normal

+++ — hyperreflexia

Clonus, which may be sustained or unsustained should be noted separately.

Hyperreflexia and clonus are indicative of an upper motor neurone spastic paralysis. The Babinski sign (a superficial reflex), which is elicited by stroking the lateral, volar aspect of the foot, is considered indicative of an upper motor neurone lesion if the great toe extends (with or without fanning of the other toes). Flexion of the great toe (and other toes) may be regarded as normal, but it must be considered in the clinical context.

It is also important to assess whether movement is voluntary, or involuntary as in an upper motor neurone spastic paralysis.

Co-ordination

Tests of co-ordination in the lower limb include the heel to the opposite shin test. This may be associated with upper limb co-ordination such as intention tremor and past pointing, as well as the ability to perform rapidly alternating movements of the feet (such as tapping the sole of the foot against the examiner's hand), the inco-ordination of which is known as dysdiadochokynesia.

Peripheral Nerve Lesions

Lateral cutaneous nerve of the thigh

Damage to this nerve (Ll spinal nerve root), usually occurs as the nerve passes medial to the anterior superior iliac spine. This will cause numbness and often hyper-aesthesia of the outer side of the thigh, known as meralgia paresthetica. There is usually localised tenderness over the nerve as it passes just medial and deep to the iliac spine.

Femoral nerve

Damage to the femoral nerve in the upper thigh may lead to paralysis of the quadriceps muscles. Irritation of the femoral nerve can be assessed by flexing the knee with the patient face down and the hip extended. This is called the femoral nerve stretch test.

Sciatic nerve

Sciatic nerve irritation is usually due to a prolapsed disc at the L4,5 or L5, Sl levels. This will press on the L5 or Sl nerve roots respectively. There will be weakness of foot dorsiflexion in the case of an L5 lesion and diminution or absence of the ankle jerk, together with weakness of plantarflexion in the case of S1 nerve root compression.

The straight leg raising test on the affected side may be markedly limited in sciatic nerve irritation. In addition, with the knee extended and the hip flexed as far as possible, passive dorsiflexion of the foot (Laseques' test) will stretch the sciatic nerve further producing pain and muscle spasm. This effect can also be obtained by flexing the neck on to the chest when the leg is raised with the knee fully extended. Sensory loss may involve a part or the whole leg below the knee. Complete sciatic nerve division, usually in the buttocks or upper thigh, will lead to total paralysis of the muscles below the knee, as well as complete sensory loss.

Common peroneal nerve

This is often damaged during dislocation of the knee, with rupture of the lateral collateral ligament of the knee or fractures of the upper fibula as the common peroneal nerve wraps around the neck of the fibula. Damage to the entire nerve will lead to complete paralysis of dorsi-flexion of the foot and ankle, while paralysis of the deep branch innervating the peroneal muscles will only produce an inversion deformity of the foot. In addition, there will often be sensory loss over the medial two-thirds of the dorsum of the foot and lateral side of the leg.

Tibial nerve

Damage to the medial popliteal nerve is usually due to a dislocation of the knee and leads to variable paralysis of plantarflexion of the foot and toes. There will also be numbness of the heel and part of the sole, the lateral side of the foot and posterior aspect of the leg. The nerve may also be compressed in the fascial tunnel behind the medial malleolus and this can lead to weakness of the intrinsic muscles of the foot.

Peripheral Nerve Lesions

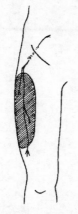

Meralgia paresthetica

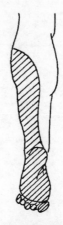

Complete sciatic nerve lesion — sensory deficit

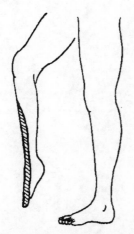

Common peroneal nerve lesion — sensory deficit and foot drop

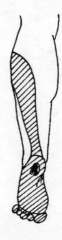

Tibial nerve lesion — sensory deficit

A Simple Guide to Orthopaedics

Chapter 5

Investigations

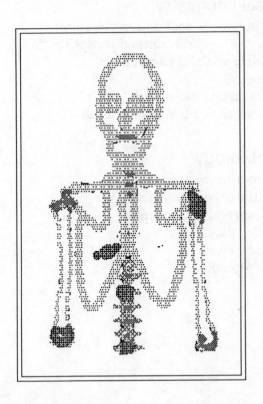

Classification

Haematology

Full blood count and blood film
Erythrocyte sedimentation rate (ESR)
Serology
Bone marrow biopsy

Clinical chemistry

Electrolytes — sodium and potassium
      calcium and phosphate
Alkaline and acid phosphatase
Urinalysis
Uric acid and cholesterol
Oxygen and carbon dioxide levels

Microbiology

Microurine and urine culture
Culture of bone and joint
Sputum and stool samples
Wound swab
Blood culture
Joint aspiration

Imaging techniques

Ultrasound
X-rays
Computerised tomography (CT)
Magnetic resonance imaging (MRI)
Nuclear scanning
Real-time imaging techniques

Histology and cytology

Needle aspiration
Trephine biopsy
Open biopsy

Miscellaneous investigations

Arthroscopy
Electrical tests
Spirometry
Exercise tolerance
Triple histamine response
Doppler ultrasound
Angiogram, venogram and lymphangiogram

Haematology

Full blood count and blood film

A full blood count (FBC) usually includes haemoglobin levels, red cell, white cell, and platelet numbers, as well as several other investigations.

In all cases of suspected infection and inflammation a white cell count (WBC) should be carried out. In pyogenic infections a neutrophilia will usually be present. The white blood cell count is usually normal in inflammatory conditions such as rheumatoid arthritis. It is only slightly elevated or normal in trauma which may otherwise mimic infection. Occasionally abnormal cells may be present, such as in the leukaemias and HIV infection.

The haemoglobin (Hb) should be assessed before any major surgery and should be a routine investigation in all major conditions.

ESR

The erythrocyte sedimentation rate (ESR) is raised in infections, in acute rheumatoid arthritis and in many other acute conditions. It is usually normal in chronic conditions such as osteoarthritis and in minor fractures.

Serology

Plasma proteins and electrophoresis

The albumin/globulin ratio is reversed in multiple myeloma, and the electrophoretic pattern is altered.

Agglutinins

The Widal test is used for typhoid fever and other salmonella infections. Brucella agglutinins may remain raised years after the patient has recovered from the original infection. Rheumatoid and latex agglutination is often raised in rheumatoid arthritis as C-reactive protein.

Haematology

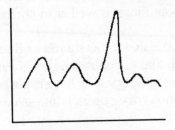

Electrophoresis

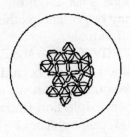

Haemagglutination

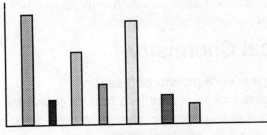

Biochemistry

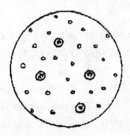

High power field of blood film

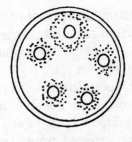

Agar plate with antibiotic sensitivity discs

HLA-B27 is usually present in 95% of patients with ankylosing spondylitis and Reiter's syndrome. This test alone is *not* diagnostic, however, as this genetic marker may be present in other conditions as well as in normal individuals.

HIV infection should be tested for as should agglutination tests for hepatitis B and C before surgery is carried out in all patients whose lifestyle may have exposed them to infection. (Intravenous drug users, homosexuals and haemophiliacs.)

Bone marrow biopsy

A biopsy of the marrow of the iliac crest or sternum is carried out in blood disorders such as multiple myeloma and lymphatic or myeloid leukaemias.

Clinical Chemistry

Electrolytes: sodium and potassium

A low potassium level may lead to a profound fall in blood pressure and retention of sodium may lead to hypernatraemia. Cardiac dysrhythmia is common in disturbances of the sodium and potassium ion levels in the serum.

Calcium and phosphate

Calcium and phosphorus levels may be altered in rickets. This helps differentiate the various types of rickets (see Chapter 12).

Hypercalcaemia is a complication of excessive bone destruction or metabolism in conditions such as secondary deposits in bone and Paget's disease. It can be lethal if not corrected prior to surgery.

Alkaline and acid phosphatase

The alkaline phosphatase is raised in conditions where there is excessive bone destruction such as in multiple secondary deposits. It is also raised in other conditions such as multiple myelomatosis and Paget's disease.

The acid phosphatase is raised in carcinoma of the prostate, which commonly metastasises to bone.

Urinalysis

Albumin may be present in the urine in renal failure and in urinary infections. The specific protein, Bence–Jones protein, is positive in about 40% of cases of multiple myeloma. Bence–Jones protein appears as a cloudiness in the urine on heating which disappears on boiling, unlike albumin which remains coagulated on boiling.

A test for *glucose* in the urine should also be routine before all orthopaedic operations. Diabetes may lead to peripheral neuritis and also to poor healing of wounds and occasionally gangrene, particularly in the lower limb, if the glucose level is not rectified.

Assessment of the pH of the urine may be useful in assessing the likely causative organism in urinary tract infection. Part of the treatment of urinary infection may be to change the pH of the urine.

Increased excretion of calcium and phosphorus may occur in rickets and other conditions where bone destruction is increased or renal absorption decreased.

Specific tests in rare congenital conditions include urinary alpha-fetoprotein in pregnant women with a foetus with spina bifida (also in the amniotic fluid) and urinary creatine phosphokinase in pseudohypertrophic muscular dystrophy.

Uric acid and cholesterol

The serum uric acid level is raised in gout. It is an essential investigation if there is any doubt that the arthritis may be gout.

The serum cholesterol is raised (hypercholesterolaemia) in many patients with ischaemic heart disease.

Oxygen and carbon dioxide levels

Oxygen and carbon dioxide saturation levels are essential in assessment of the severely injured patient.

Microbiology Investigations

Microurine

The urine should always be inspected for cloudiness and for blood. The odour should also be noted.

The urine should be examined microscopically for blood and pus cells and then centrifuged and the sediment examined for bacteria.

If urinary infection is suspected, the urine should be cultured and the sensitivity to antibiotics of any bacteria grown should be determined. This will take 2–3 days.

Culture of bone and joint

In conditions where an unusual infection of bone or joint is suspected, such as tuberculosis, a culture for the tubercle bacillus should be performed. This may take 3–6 weeks. If an anaerobic organism such as Clostridium welchii (which causes gas gangrene) is suspected, anaerobic culture will be necessary.

Sputum and stool samples

In suspected tuberculosis of bones and joints the sputum should be cultured for the tubercle bacillus and examined under the microscope for acid fast bacilli.

Microbiology Investigations

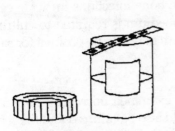

Urine analysis

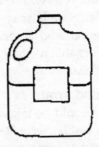

24hr urine collection for
Bence–Jones protein

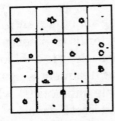

Cell counts using
counting chamber

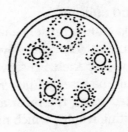

Agar plate with antibiotic
sensitivity discs

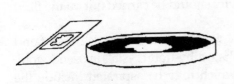

Tuberculosis:
Zeil–Nielsen
stain and culture

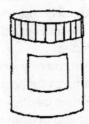

Stool sample for
microscopy and culture

If secondary deposits in bone are suspected to have arisen from a lung carcinoma, sputum cytology for malignant cells will be required.

Salmonella may cause bone infections in sickle cell anaemia, and a specific medium is required to culture this organism. Stool culture may also be positive for salmonella.

Wound swab

Pus should be taken and examined microscopically for cells and bacteria. It should also be cultured and the sensitivity of any bacteria determined. Pus for microscopy and culture should be taken *before* the wound is cleaned with an antiseptic and before antibiotics are given.

Blood culture

Blood culture must be taken before antibiotics are given if acute osteomyelitis, pyogenic arthritis or other infection is suspected. Sensitivity of the bacteria to antibiotics should be assessed but *intravenous* treatment is usually started using the most appropriate antibiotic(s) while awaiting results, which may take at least 2 days.

Joint aspiration

In suspected joint infections such as pyogenic arthritis of the knee, the joint should be aspirated with a fairly fine needle. Microscopy, including a gram stain for organisms, culture and sensitivity should be carried out on the fluid obtained.

Microscopy will show uric acid crystals in gout and calcium pyrophosphate dihydrate crystals in pseudogout.

Other cavities which may be aspirated include the chest and abdomen. Abscesses may also be aspirated to obtain pus for gram stain, culture and sensitivity.

Where gas gangrene is suspected, microscopy, as well as culture for anaerobic organisms, should be carried out. In revision operations routine culture, sensitivity and microscopy should be performed at the time of re-operation.

Imaging Techniques

Imaging techniques include X-rays, nuclear scanning, computerised tomography (CT) and magnetic resonance imaging (MRI) as well as ultrasound for soft tissue visualisation. This specialty has expanded considerably in recent years and has improved the investigation of orthopaedic conditions. Three dimensional and subtraction CT and MRI scanning are amongst the latest techniques for visualisation particularly in tumours, surgery and trauma where indicated.

A standard chest X-ray with posterior/anterior and lateral views is sufficient for diagnosing most chest conditions. In the case of tumours with possible secondary deposits, CT scanning of the chest may be necessary in addition to a plain X-ray.

Standard bone and joint X-rays are sufficient in most cases.

Ultrasound

Ultrasound is a simple diagnostic method which does not irradiate or harm the patient. It will delineate different density tissues by the use of very high frequency sound waves. Its use is relatively limited but it has a place in the diagnosis of soft tissue tumours, particularly in the abdomen, and also for conditions such as congenital dislocation of the hip.

X-rays

X-rays of affected bone and joints will often be sufficient for diagnosis. In most cases at least two views at right angles to each other, an anteroposterior (AP) and a lateral, will be required. It is important that the bone and joint above and below the lesion be X-rayed as well as the affected bone and joint or joints.

A tomogram is helpful for diagnosing a bone sequestrum in the centre of a cavity which might otherwise be obscured by the overlying bone or to confirm a non-union of a fracture. In this technique the X-ray tube is rotated so that only one part of the bone is in focus at a time.

Chest X-rays

A chest X-ray is essential in all patients in whom a tumour is suspected, and also in all patients, particularly over the age of 50, who may require a major operation. This is also important in all patients who have a history of chest problems, and particularly in suspected tuberculosis of bones and joints where a primary focus in the lung may be responsible. A chest X-ray is also important in suspected malignant tumours with possible pulmonary secondaries.

Contrast media

Injection of contrast media into joints and cavities may help outline difficult areas. This includes air contrast arthrograms in knees and other joints. Injections of dye (radiopaque contrast medium) into sinuses may help delineate the extent of the sinus cavity or abscesses.

A radiopaque contrast medium injected into the spinal cavity is called a myelogram. This will show not only a tumour blocking the spinal canal but also protrusion of discs causing pressure on nerve roots in conditions such

Organic Imaging

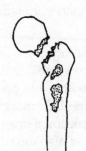

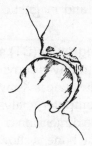

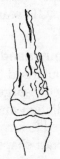

X-ray appearance of a pathological fracture

X-ray appearance of an arthritic hip

Tomogram

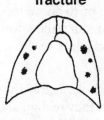

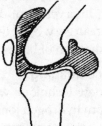

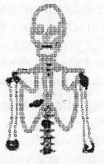

Chest X-ray

Arthrogram

Nuclear medicine

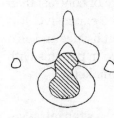

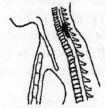

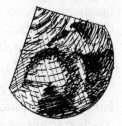

CT scan

Magnetic resonance imaging

Ultrasound

as sciatica and low back pain. Myelograms are now being superseded in many cases by computerised tomography (CT) scanning and magnetic resonance imaging (MRI).

Computerised tomography (CT) scanning

Computerised tomography is proving invaluable in orthopaedic surgery. The bone is X-rayed with a low dose of radiation and a computer analyses the information received to form a two dimension cross-sectional image. The exact shape of the bone is shown and also the soft tissues overlying the bone, revealing the extent of spread of tumours or infections into the soft tissues. It is more expensive than a simple X-ray, and is therefore not done routinely except where it will be of particular value, such as in prolapse of an intervertebral disc or to show the exact site for tumour surgery. New techniques allow for 3-dimensional visualisation of bones and joints.

Magnetic resonance imaging

This is a relatively new technique which measures the radiation emitted from hydrogen ions as they realign after being oriented in a strong magnetic field. There is no ionising radiation used. This is particularly useful in the diagnosis of soft tissue lesions, such as ruptures of knee ligaments, since it gives a greater range of contrast than CT scanning, but at present is far more expensive. It is particularly valuable for visualising soft tissues and also in tumour surgery. It should not be used in patients with ferrous metal implants or cardiac pacemakers.

Nuclear scanning

Nuclear scanning in orthopaedics involves the intra- venous injection of a radio-isotope, technetium-99m methylene diphosphonate, which selectively binds to bony tissue. The concentration of the isotope is partially determined by the vascularity of the tissue involved. Hence in the presence of a normally growing epiphysis, bony infection or neoplasia, there will be greater uptake. The suspected area of pathology, and often the whole patient, will be scanned by a gamma-camera, which detects the level of emission. Regions of high concentration are commonly referred to as 'hot' areas.

In most patients the kidney and bladder will also show pooling of this isotope which is excreted through the renal tract, it will make these viscera appear hot.

Another isotope commonly used in orthopaedics is gallium. Gallium scanning is used to detect foci of inflammation, and some neoplastic tissues as a result of its affinity for chronic inflammatory cells.

Other imaging techniques

Other imaging techniques include *cineradiography, fluroscopy,* or *videotaping.* Cineradiography, unlike fluroscopy provides a permanent record of active movement, and with higher resolution than is possible with videotape. Pathology, that is not immediately obvious on standard plain X-rays, may become apparent when movement is displayed. It may also be retained for future reference and comparison.

Other uses of videotaping include gait analysis, and recording of operative procedures (particularly arthroscopy) for instruction and future reference.

Histology and Cytology

Needle aspiration

Aspiration biopsy is useful, not only in infections, but also in certain tumours. This applies particularly to soft tissue tumours and in some bony tumours. The aspirate is also cultured if there is any possibility of infection.

Trephine biopsy

Trephine biopsy of bones is indicated in suspected primary tumours and particularly in secondary deposits. The trephine is a wide-bored needle of about 2–3 mm diameter with a cutting edge. The core of tumour is approximately 10–30 mm in length and 2 mm in diameter. The core is rubbed across one or two glass slides and the remainder is sent for pathology. If there is any possibility of infection the specimen should also be sent for gram staining and culture. The trephine biopsy is particularly valuable for biopsy of inaccessible sites such as the lumbar spine.

Open biopsy

If a larger biopsy is needed an open biopsy is carried out. A wedge of tumour, including the bone and if possible the edge of the tumour, is removed. In certain tumours, such as osteochondroma, the *whole* tumour should be excised as it may not be obvious which part of the tumour may be undergoing malignant change. A provisional diagnosis can sometimes be made on examination of the smear on the slide. A definitive diagnosis will usually mean a wait of several days while bone and cartilage is decalcified.

No major operation should be carried out, particularly for primary tumours, until a biopsy result is availa-

Biopsy and Aspiration

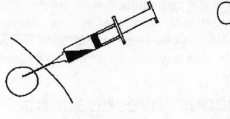

Fine needle biopsy

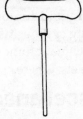

Trephine biopsy

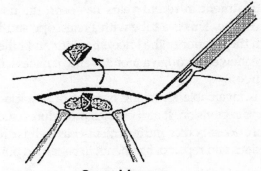

Open biopsy

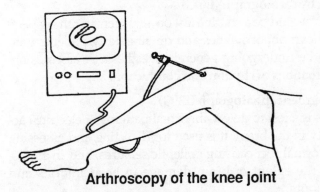

Arthroscopy of the knee joint

ble, as occasionally an infection or other condition may mimic a tumour, and vice versa. Examples are Ewing's sarcoma of bone which may mimic osteomyelitis, and a parathyroid tumour with associated hypercalcaemia causing cystic areas in bones. These may mimic a primary malignant tumour or a secondary deposit from carcinoma elsewhere.

Miscellaneous Investigations

Arthroscopy

One of the most significant advances in both diagnosis and treatment in recent years has been the use of the arthroscope. This is a tube with a telescope and light by which the interior of the knee, shoulder and other joints can be viewed through a monitor and, if necessary, operated upon.

It is invaluable for taking biopsies of suspicious areas under direct vision. It also enables procedures, such as removal of loose bodies and torn menisci, as well as division of adhesions and repair of ligaments, to be carried out.

Electrical tests

Electrocardiograph (ECG)

This should be a routine test on all patients with suspected heart abnormalities and on all elderly patients who will be undergoing general anaesthesia. It assesses abnormalities of rhythm and conduction.

Electroencephalograph (EEG)

This is a test to detect abnormal patterns of electrical activity in the brain. It is used for detecting and assessing abnormal foci causing epileptic seizures, and in assessing the extent of brain damage in head injuries and tumours.

Electromyography (EMG)

In this test a needle electrode is placed in a muscle to assess electrical activity and this is displayed on an oscilloscope. Axonal degeneration in a muscle with denervation will be represented by 'fibrillation potentials' instead of being 'silent' as occurs in the normal resting muscle with an intact nerve supply. This indicates disruption of muscle innervation but may not appear until 3 weeks after the interruption of neural conduction. Peripheral neuropathies and anterior horn involvement in the spinal cord have a different appearance from denervated muscles.

Nerve conduction studies

Conduction velocity is measured using surface electrodes. It varies with the age of the patient and room temperature. Normal conduction velocity is approximately about 45 metres per second in the lower limb and 50 metres per second in the arm. Damage to a nerve and its myelin sheath will slow or completely block conduction through an injured segment of the nerve. A generalised abnormality is indicative of a peripheral neuropathy while a localised lesion is indicative of a single nerve injury. Nerve conduction studies on sensory nerves are easier to perform than those on motor nerves. Lesions of the central nervous system do not produce abnormalities in peripheral nerve conduction studies.

Spirometry

The vital capacity and other measures of lung function can be of value to the anaesthetist, especially in assessing elderly patients with poor respiratory function.

Exercise tolerance

In elderly patients assessment of exercise tolerance and

its effects on the ECG, pulse and blood pressure, may be of value in assessing the likely effects of increased mobility following hip or knee replacement. Graded increasing workload on an exercise bicycle (eg. Bruce or de Brusk protocol) or treadmill will allow accurate assessment of an exercising 'stationary' patient.

Triple histamine response

This is a test used mainly in brachial plexus injuries to assess the level of division. In a very high lesion at the cord level proximal to the posterior root axon, injection of a drop of histamine into the forearm will cause a reflex vasodilatation with a weal and hyperaemia. If the division is distal to the axon no reflex can take place and there will be no 'triple response'.

Doppler ultrasound

This is particularly useful in the lower limb to assess blood flow over an artery by means of an ultrasound probe. This can accurately show the site of a block or narrowing in an artery, and as a result, often avoid the need for an angiogram.

Angiogram, venogram and lymphangiogram

This is an X-ray of the arterial tree after injection of a radiopaque dye into a major vessel. The arterial tree, together with any occlusion or narrowing, can be demonstrated. More sophisticated techniques include digital subtraction angiography where a computer is able to eliminate soft tissue and bone from the image.

A venogram is the injection of a radiopaque dye into a major vein to demonstrate venous occlusion in patients suspected of having a deep vein thrombosis. The injection of a contrast medium into lymphatics, or lyphangiogram, may be indicated in lymphatic obstuction.

Chapter 6

Treatment

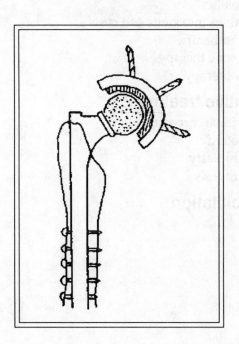

Classification

Conservative treatment
Physiotherapy
Supports

Medical treatment
Analgesia
Anti-inflammatory medication
Antibiotics
Injections into joints and cysts
Chemotherapy
Hormone therapy
Radiotherapy

Operative treatment
Soft tissue correction
Osteotomy
Arthroplasty
Arthrodesis

Rehabilitation

Conservative Treatment

Physiotherapy

Physiotherapy can be divided into three main categories:

Thermal and cryotherapy

Radiant or superficial heat are suitable for patients who are unfit to travel to a physiotherapy department or who have an implanted prosthesis. Sometimes ice packs are used if there is considerable bruising immediately after injury.

Deep heat, such as short wave diathermy or ultrasound can be used in cases where there is *no* implanted prosthesis or plates, nails or screws.

Massage

Massage in its various forms is soothing to the patient but has a limited place.

Exercise

Exercise may be active or passive. Active exercises, where the patient exercises the joint, are by far the most valuable. They increase the power of muscles and actively move the joints, often increasing both the range of joint movement and joint lubrication.

Passive exercises, where the physiotherapist moves the joints, may be necessary where the joint is paralysed or where the patient is reluctant to move the limb. They have a place, but are of much less value than active exercise. They are useful, however, in preventing contractures across joints, particularly in the shoulder, hand and knee.

In addition to passive exercises performed by the physiotherapist, a machine called a continuous passive motion machine (CPM) is now in use. This machine is powered by an electric motor and is used mainly on the lower limb and occasionally on the upper limb. It moves the limb through a variable range of movements at a pre-determined speed. It is invaluable for patients recovering from severe knee or hip operations (and occasionally the upper limb) to prevent the joints from becoming stiff postoperatively.

It has also been shown that constant movement by these machines markedly improves the nutrition of the joint cartilage and often accelerates the recovery of joint mobility.

Transcutaneous electrical nerve stimulation (TENS)
In chronic pain, particularly low back pain and sciatica, transcutaneous nerve stimulation with a battery powered machine worn by the patient may relieve pain. A small pad placed over the site of maximum tenderness on the skin can electrically stimulate the underlying cutaneous nerves in differing amplitude and duration.

Supports

Boots and innersoles
In the case of a short leg, a contracted knee or an equinus ankle, a raise on a boot, either on the heel alone or on both the sole and the heel, may be necessary.

Many other supports are in common use, including innersoles in shoes to support 'fallen arches' and soft plastic inserts to relieve pressure areas on the sole of the foot particularly the heel (plantar fasciitis) and forefoot (anterior metatarsalgia).

Calipers
A caliper is a metal support for an unstable foot, knee or occasionally hip. It consists merely of one or two metal side arms, usually attached to a boot or shoe. In patients with weak dorsiflexion of the foot, it may be combined

Physiotherapy

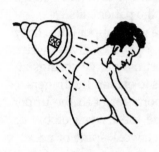

Radiant heat

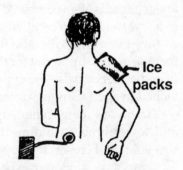

Ice packs

Transcutaneous electrical nerve stimulation (TENS)

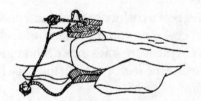

Short wave ultrasound diathermy

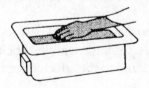

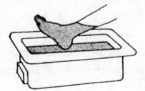

Wax baths

with either a spring or a back stop to prevent the foot going into equinus when the patient walks. In patients with weak knees, the caliper must extend above the knee to support it and prevent it from collapsing. The above-knee caliper is often combined with a knee bending hinge to allow the knee to bend when the patient sits.

Supports can also be used for a weak upper limb. They include a 'cock-up' splint for the support of a weak wrist. In radial nerve palsy the support may have springs attached to special finger supports to extend the fingers.

There are many other supports for both the upper and lower limb, including those for a weak elbow or shoulder, and corsets to support a weak spine or neck.

Temporary supports can be made out of plaster of Paris or various plastics and include supports for the knee, ankle and upper limb.

Bed supports

These include special cushions to support a patient's back, supports and cushions under the sacrum and under the heels to prevent pressure sores in bed, and pillows under the legs to elevate the feet or to keep the knee flexed after a hip operation.

Walking aids

A variety of crutches is available. Some allow the patient to bear weight mainly on the shoulders and hands. In addition there are short elbow crutches and walking frames.

Walking sticks vary from those with a broad base and four prongs, called quadrapods, to single walking sticks which are used in the *opposite* hand to the affected leg.

Exercises
Upper limb

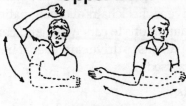

Shoulder

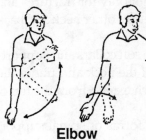

Elbow

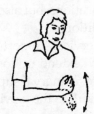

Wrist

Lower limb

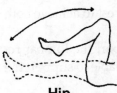

Hip

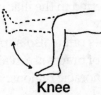

Knee

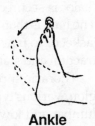

Ankle

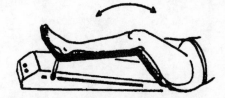

Continuous passive movement machine

Wheelchairs and motorised vehicles

A variety of wheelchairs is available, from ordinary wheelchairs where the patient is self propelled, to electric or petrol driven wheelchairs allowing patients on the road. Special adaptations to cars with hand controls will allow disabled patients to drive cars, even if both legs are completely paralysed.

Spinal supports

These include supports for the cervical, thoracic and lumbar regions and are used not only for fractures and dislocations, but also for a variety of other neck and back conditions.

Cervical supports vary from soft collars and supports which extend up to the back of the neck and under the jaw to 'Minerva' supports which extend from the top of the skull to the pelvis.

Other less commonly used forms of spinal support include halo-thoracic and halo-pelvic traction. A metal 'halo' is secured by pins to the outer table of the skull. The halo is then attached by distraction rods to a plaster jacket or to pins inserted in the iliac crest to achieve both traction and stability.

Thoracic supports often also support the lumbar region. Various types of braces are available to support the lumbar and lower thoracic regions.

Supports

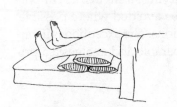

Three pillows

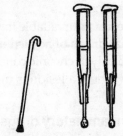

Canes and crutches

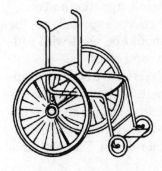

Wheelchair

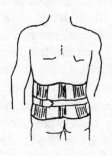

Spinal support

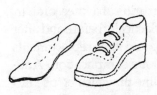

Inner sole and raised boot

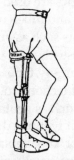

Above knee caliper

Medical Treatment

Analgesics

Analgesics are available in varying strengths. It is important that drugs of addiction be avoided where possible, particularly in chronic conditions. The exception is in oncology where a lesion is inoperable and analgesia a priority.

Anti-inflammatory drugs

Non-steroidal anti-inflammatory drugs, such as ibuprofen and diclofenac, are used commonly for arthritis. They have some effect in diminishing inflammation and oedema. All these drugs have side effects, especially on the gastrointestinal system, and should be used with caution and for a limited period in most cases.

Aspirin has been shown to be effective both as an analgesic and as an anti-inflammatory drug but also has side effects. Steroids such as hydrocortisone and prednisone are sometimes used in advanced rheumatoid arthritis, as are gold salts and other drugs. These all have potentially severe side effects.

Antibiotics

Antibiotics are used for specific infections such as osteomyelitis and tuberculosis. They are occasionally injected into joints such as in pyogenic arthritis of a knee joint. In many cases they are used prophylactically before and after major surgery, for example in hip and knee replacements where infection would be a serious complication. Antibiotics such as gentamicin in saline may also be used to wash out wounds during major operations such as a total hip or knee replacement. In addition, systemic antibiotics are usually given in large doses at the time of op-

Medical Treatment

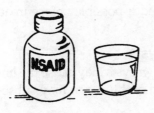

Analgesics and anti-inflammatory drugs

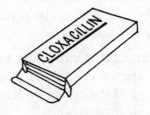

Antibiotics

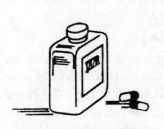

Chemotherapy and hormones

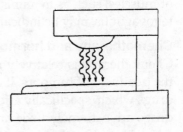

Radiotherapy

eration and then continued for at least three days post-operatively. In the case of suspected infection, treatment may be continued for one to three weeks and even up to three months or longer. It is important, however, that the appropriate antibiotic be given for the infection being treated. In all infections it is important that the sensitivity of the organism be determined if possible before treatment is started.

Injections into joints and cysts

Injection of cortisone into *benign* cysts may cause the lining of the cyst to be absorbed and the cyst may subsequently resolve.

Antibiotics may be injected into joints for acute joint infections. Drainage with a suction drain, plus large doses of intravenous antibiotics, is the usual treatment.

Occasionally there is a place for the injection of hydrocortisone into joints such as the knee in osteoarthritis or rheumatoid arthritis. This carries, however, the potential danger of steroid arthropathy.

Injection of steroids into chronic tender partial tears of muscles, such as in tennis elbow or in de Quervain's tenovaginitis, may be indicated.

Chemotherapy and hormones

Chemotherapy is relatively new and is used mainly in the treatment of tumours. It consists of a variety of new drugs which specifically affect proliferating cells. These drugs are extremely toxic and the patient may require other drugs after the chemotherapy to undo their harmful effects on healthy tissues.

Drugs currently in use include methotrexate, vincristine, cisplatin and doxorubicin hydrochloride. These drugs are given intravenously in various combinations,

Medical Treatment

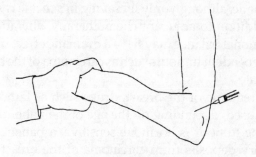

**Cortisone injection
for tennis elbow**

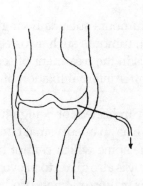

**Drainage of septic
arthritis**

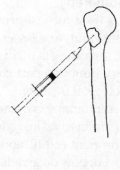

**Cortisone injection into
benign bone cyst**

usually for a period of up to two years, and usually about every three weeks for approximately three days.

The effects of these drugs on tumours such as Ewing's sarcoma and occasionally osteogenic sarcoma can be dramatic, although only lifesaving in specific cases.

In addition to adjuvant chemotherapy, alteration of the hormonal balance may have a dramatic effect in hormone dependent tumours such as carcinoma of the breast or prostate.

In carcinoma of the breast, drugs such as tamoxifen may be used, depending on the age of the patient. Provided the tumour is hormone sensitive, a patient with secondary deposits from carcinoma of the breast may survive for many years, even following pathological fractures.

In carcinoma of the prostate there is occasionally a place for orchidectomy. The administration of stilboestrol may also have a beneficial effect.

Radiotherapy

This is used for fast-growing tumours such as Ewing's sarcoma and, to a lesser extent, tumours such as osteogenic sarcoma. Its main place is in the treatment of secondary tumours, particularly after internal fixation of a pathological fracture.

Radiotherapy is occasionally indicated for benign tumours in inaccessible sites, such as an aneurysmal bone cyst or giant cell tumour of the spine which cannot be removed. Low dose radiotherapy is also given to prevent recurrence of myositis ossificans in those patients predisposed to this complication, for example following major hip surgery in patients with previous ossification.

Operative treatment

Soft tissue correction

There is a place for soft tissue correction in contractures of joints in poliomyelitis or spastic paralysis, including flexion contractures of the hip, knee or ankle. This procedure performed by either open or closed methods, can often correct a deformity, allow realignment of the joint and permit the patient to be weight-bearing. Soft tissue correction may be combined with bony correction.

In constriction of tendon sheaths such as the flexor sheath of the fingers (trigger finger) or over the radial styloid process (de Quervain's syndrome), division of the tendon sheaths alone will often free the constricted area.

Similarly, neurolysis of nerves such as the median nerve under the carpal tunnel in the wrist will allow for recovery of a sensory and motor deficit.

In rheumatoid arthritis proliferation of synovium may cause erosion of the cartilage if left untreated. Excision of synovium, particularly of the metacarpophalangeal joints of the fingers, and in the knee, may delay the erosion and degeneration.

In partial paralysis with muscle imbalance, transfer of working tendons may partially compensate for paralysis. An example is the transfer of the tibialis posterior tendon from being an inverter and plantar-flexor of the foot to being a dorsiflexor of the ankle and foot. Tendon transfers around the wrist and hands can compensate for imbalanced weakness in nerve injuries and paralysis, provided there is adequate power of at least grade 4 in the tendon to be transferred and provided any deformities are first corrected.

Osteotomy

An osteotomy is realignment by removing or opening out a wedge of bone in order to correct a deformity. This will not only correct a deformity such as a flexed, valgus or varus knee, but also allows a different and healthier area of cartilage to accept weight-bearing. Osteotomy can also diminish the excessive blood supply to an inflamed or arthritic area of the joint and allow oedema to subside. Osteotomy is, however, usually palliative rather than curative as the original area of osteoarthritis or degeneration is not replaced. Osteotomy of bone will also correct malalignment in malunited fractures and so prevent the onset of osteoarthritis due to asymmetrical pressure on a joint.

Osteotomy of the trochanteric region of the hip corrects an adduction or abduction deformity and allows a different area of the cartilage on the head of the femur to be weight-bearing. It also decreases excessive hyperaemia and oedema of the joint capsule.

A varus deformity of the knee may be associated with narrowing and osteoarthritis of the medial joint compartment with sparing of the lateral compartment. A lateral wedge of 20°–30° in the upper tibia will change the weight-bearing of the tibia from varus to valgus. The good lateral compartment will then take most of the body weight and regeneration of part of the medial articular cartilage may then occur.

Osteotomies of bone are usually held by nails, plates or staples.

Arthroplasties

An arthroplasty is the formation of a movable, mobile joint from a stiff joint, usually by joint replacement. It can be divided into three main types.

Operative Treatment

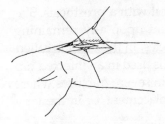

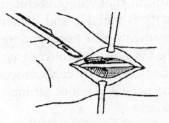

De Quervains syndrome — division of tendon sheath

Carpal tunnel syndrome — division of flexor retinaculum

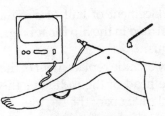

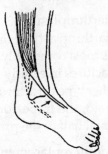

Arthroscopic synovectomy

Tendon transfer

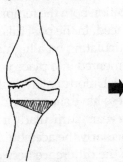

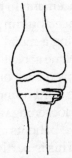

X-ray appearance of a genu varum deformity

X-ray appearance of a corrective osteotomy

Excision arthroplasty

An excision arthroplasty is the excision of a destroyed or painful joint without replacing it with a prosthesis. Stability is variable and dependent upon any remaining ligaments, scar tissue and muscles. In the hip it is called the Girdlestone arthroplasty. It is used in an infected hip after a failed hip replacement, in severe fractures where the patient is not fit for hip replacement, or in the very elderly.

Excision arthroplasty of part of the proximal phalanx of the big toe in hallux valgus in elderly patients (Keller's operation) or excision of the head of the radius in a severe fracture are other examples.

Hemiarthroplasty

Hemiarthroplasty is the replacement of half of a joint. This is most commonly performed in the hip for subcapital fractures in elderly patients.

Other types of arthroplasty include replacement of the scaphoid, the trapezium, the head of the radius or the proximal half of the proximal phalanx of the big toe.

Total joint replacement

The most successful total arthroplasty to date has been hip replacement. In this operation both the femoral head and the acetabulum are replaced. In the past this has entailed using a metal head articulating on a high density polyethylene socket, both cemented into place with methyl methacrylate bone cement. Unfortunately, in the past, up to one third or more of these have shown evidence of failure or loosening within ten years, particularly in young and active patients and particularly the acetabular component. This is partly due to the difference between the modulus of elasticity of the cement and that of bone as

Arthroplasty

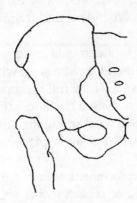

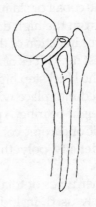

Girdlestone's excision arthroplasty

Austin–Moore hemiarthroplasty

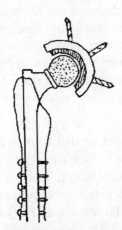

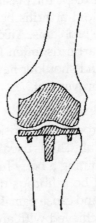

X-ray appearance of a cementless hip replacement

X-ray appearance of a total knee replacement

well as the relatively high friction of metal on high density polyethylene. Other factors are metal sensitivity to chrome cobalt or stainless steel, reactions from wear particles from the high density polyethylene and fragmentation or infection of the bone cement.

Most new types of total hip replacements are cementless. The Huckstep hip has an inert titanium stem which is locked into place with screws to allow full postoperative weight-bearing. A partially stabilised zirconium (PSZ) ceramic or chrome cobalt femoral head articulates with a high density polyethylene socket held in place with screws.

Other types of total joint replacement, which are extensively used, include total knee replacements with a metal femoral component articulating with a high density polyethylene tibial component. These are usually held in place by cement or without cement by a friction fit.

Most other arthroplasties have not proved very successful except for plastic arthroplasty of the fingers in rheumatoid arthritis but even the plastic in these may produce problems. Ankle arthroplasties, except in rheumatoid arthritis, often fail while arthroplasties of both elbow and shoulder have a limited place and need further improvement.

Arthrodesis

An arthrodesis is a fusion of a joint so that it does not move at all. This is usually achieved by excising the joint and obtaining a bony fusion. If bony fusion fails the result will be a fibrous union which will usually move slightly and cause pain if stressed. Fusion of the knee joint is best achieved with an intramedullary locking nail. A Huckstep titanium nail with locking screws is probably

Arthrodesis

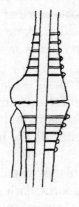

Knee

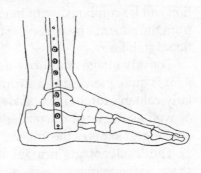

Pantalar

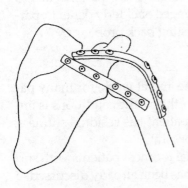

Shoulder

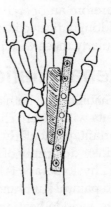

Wrist

the most satisfactory for this purpose and allows for immediate full weight-bearing.

The same applies to the use of a similar locking nail for a pantalar arthrodesis (combined ankle and subtaloid joints). In the hip and shoulder, extra-articular fixation can be combined with internal fixation. Bone graft from the patient's own iliac crest is often used as an additional stabiliser.

The advantage of a successful arthrodesis is that the joint is quite painless and strong. It is therefore particularly valuable for the knee, ankle, subtalar joints and toes, as well as the wrist or smaller joints such as the interphalangeal joints of the fingers.

The disadvantages include both lack of movement and strain on the neighbouring joints. This is particularly seen in arthrodesis of the hip where additional strain is placed on the lumbar and thoracic regions of the spine, often resulting in low back pain. Arthrodesis of the hip is therefore an operation for some young patients and is seldom indicated in middle aged or elderly patients, particularly those with pre-existing back problems.

Rehabilitation

Rehabilitation, both at home and at work, for many patients with severe chronic orthopaedic conditions is important, particularly if the patient has residual stiffness, pain or deformity of a major joint.

Physiotherapy is essential for most patients with stiff and painful joints and this has been already discussed. It may include heat and massage, but more importantly, active and occasionally passive exercises. Walking on soft sand in bare feet is good for the patient following ankle and foot operations, while cycling on an exercise bike may

Rehabilitation

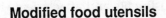

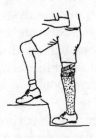
Modified food utensils

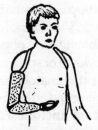
Artificial limb

Gait retraining

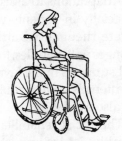
Wheelchair

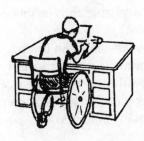
Early re-employment

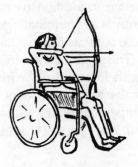
Recreation

be indicated following hip, knee and back operations. Swimming in a heated pool is the best overall exercise for orthopaedic conditions, particularly those involving the back, shoulders, hips and knees.

Rehabilitation of patients following major operations on hip, knee or spine on paraplegic patients or those with severe rheumatoid arthritis, may include considerable retraining and adjustments, both at work and in the home. This may include ramps, supporting rails and low benches together with adjustments and attachments to machines.

Adaptations to assist in the activities of daily living, especially in patients with amputations, paralysis and severe rheumatoid arthritis, may include combs and sponges with handles, towels with loops, baths with seats, and supports in the lavatory. Special attachments to eating utensils such as rubber handles on spoons and forks, are also available.

The social rehabilitation of patients with severe deformities is also important as these patients may otherwise become housebound, introspective and depressed.

Mobility for the severely disabled is particularly important. In addition to wheelchairs, cars with special hand controls and automatic gears are available, thus enabling these patients to leave their homes.

The severely disabled, if given assistance in improving their home and work environment, are particularly reliable workers. In many countries the law requires large companies to employ disabled people as up to 3% of their staff. It is essential that this is actually enforced.

Section II

Specific Orthopaedic
Conditions

Chapter 7

Congenital and Paediatric Conditions

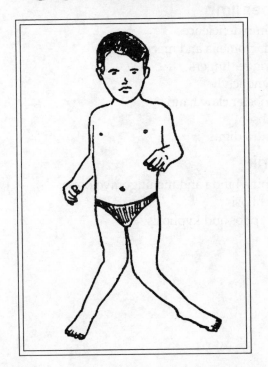

Classification

Generalised abnormalities
Achondroplasia
Osteogenesis imperfecta
Arthrogryposis
Still's disease
Hurler's syndrome
Diaphyseal aclasis
Hypothyroidism

Upper limb
Limb deficiences
Macromelia and macrodactyly
Trigger fingers
Syndactyly
Lobster claw hand
Absent
Extra digits

Trunk
Spina bifida and meningomyelocele
Scoliosis
Kyphos and kyphosis

Lower limb

Whole Limb
Phocomelia
Macrodactyly

Hip
Congenital dislocation (CDH)
Slipped epiphysis
Perthes' disease
Transient synovitis
Septic arthritis
Coxa vara and valga
Protrusio acetabuli

Knee
Genu varum and valgum
Genu recurvatum
Osteochondritis
Congenital webbing

Ankle and foot
Talipes equino varus
Talipes calcaneo valgus
Pes cavus
Pes planus
Metatarsus adductus
Osteochondritis or avascular necrosis
Exostoses
Accessory bones
Syndactyly

Introduction

Diagnosis

A clinical history is essential and can reveal a genetic abnormality which may be autosomal dominant or recessive or sex-linked. Such deformities include diaphyseal aclasis or multiple osteochondromata and achondroplasia with dwarfism. There may be a history of maternal use of drugs such as thalidomide, irradiation of the foetus in the critical first three months of development or a history of maternal rubella infection. Finally there is a large group with no known cause.

Diagnosis may be easy with evidence of a classical anomaly at birth such as differences in the size or shape of limbs or multiple abnormalities which may be symmetrical, such as microdactyly or talipes equino varus. The opposite limb must always be examined. It may show a similar deformity, which is usually painless, with no evidence that the abnormality is acquired such as operation scars. All gradations of spina bifida including a meningomyelocele must also be looked for.

Besides skeletal abnormalities, there may be other congenital abnormalities and thus a full examination should always be carried out. Other family members may show similar abnormalities or give a classic history which in most cases simplifies the diagnosis.

Relatively common non-orthopaedic abnormalities include: cleft lip and palate, Down's syndrome, cardiac abnormalities such as tetralogy of Fallot (which produces a boot shaped heart) and abdominal visceral abnormalities such as pyloric stenosis.

Diagnosis

Orthopaedic anomalies

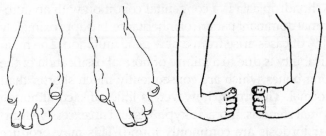

Microdactyly

Talipes equino varus

Family history

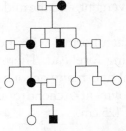

Autosomal dominant disorder

Autosomal recessive disorder

Non-orthopaedic anomalies

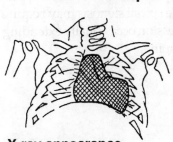

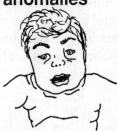

X-ray appearance of a 'boot heart'

Facial features — Hurler's syndrome

Generalised Abnormalities

Achondroplasia

Achondroplasia is a congenital condition with an autosomal dominant pattern of inheritance, but approximately 80% of cases arise from a new gene mutation. The main disability is due to a failure of normal ossification of the long bones which are consequently much shorter than normal. The trunk, however, is little affected although spinal stenosis, thoracic kyphosis and an excessive lumbar lordosis are commonly found. This may produce severe neurological sequelae such as spinal cord compression and even quadriplegia.

The hands are broad, quite divergent, and the middle three fingers of equal length.

The head is slightly larger than normal with a depressed nasal bridge and bulging forehead. There is, however, no mental impairment and many achondroplastic dwarfs find gainful employment. Achondroplastic dwarfs are seldom taller than 125 cm.

Treatment

The complications of achondroplasia include degenerative joint disease, especially osteoarthritis of the hips, which may require joint replacement. Nerve compression and paralysis due to the spinal stenosis may require laminectomy and decompression occasionally extending for the entire length of the spine.

Generalised Abnormalities

Achondroplasia

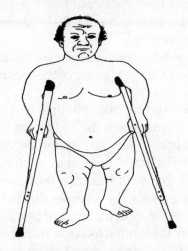

**Achondroplastic dwarf — may
occasionally require crutches
as paresis or paralysis may
result from spinal stenosis**

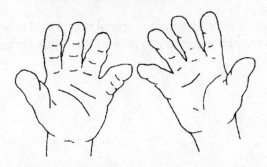

Hands of an achondroplastic dwarf

Osteogenesis imperfecta

(Fragilitas ossium)

Osteogenesis imperfecta is usually inherited as an auto-somal dominant trait. As a result of defective collagen synthesis, the bones are abnormally brittle and multiple fractures are common.

Other collagen-containing tissues such as the tendons, ligaments, skin, teeth and sclerae of the eyes may also be affected.

All gradations occur, from multiple fractures at birth to less severe forms where the child does not develop fractures until later in life. The sclerae, especially in the late-manifesting or 'tarda' cases, may be blue due to lack of opaque collagen with resulting translucency to the choroid. There may also be deafness due to otosclerosis and ligamentous laxity in the chain of ossicles.

As a result of these often multiple fractures, the limbs and trunk may be deformed and shortened. Fractures should be treated by the standard methods and usually heal satisfactorily. The remaining multiple deformities, however, especially of the femur, may require internal fixation including intramedullary nailing, to straighten them.

In severe cases calipers, spinal braces and other supports may be necessary to protect the brittle bones.

Generalised Abnormalities

Osteogenesis imperfecta

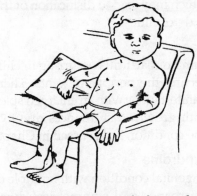

Child with osteogenesis imperfecta showing limbs with multiple deformities

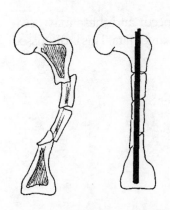

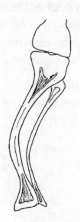

X-ray appearance of a deformed femur with multiple fractures

X-ray appearance of a deformed tibia

Arthrogryposis

This is due to collagen replacement of muscles surrounding joints and there are often multiple flexion contractures with thickened joint capsules and severe deformities which may lead to dislocation of the joints and very severe deformities.

Still's disease

This is rheumatoid arthritis occurring in childhood and mainly affecting the peripheral joints. There are often systemic manifestations with an enlarged spleen and liver together with growth disturbances due to epiphyseal damage. The condition is discussed in Chapter 10.

Hurler's syndrome

This is a congenital condition with multiple deformities, mental disturbance and symmetrical dwarfism with limbs and trunk equally affected. It is due to a rare mucopolysaccharide disorder.

Diaphyseal aclasis

Multiple osteochondromata occur and these may occasionally develop into chondrosarcomata. This is discussed further in Chapter 8.

Other tumours

These are discussed in Chapter 8.

Generalised Abnormalities

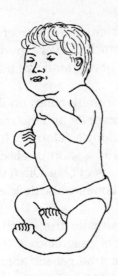

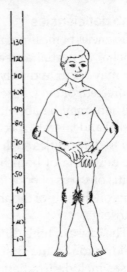

**Arthrogryposis
multiplex congenita**

Still's disease

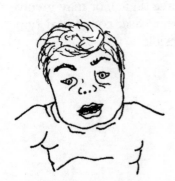

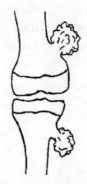

Hurler's syndrome

**X-ray appearance of
diaphyseal aclasis**

Upper Limb Conditions

Limb deficiencies

Deficiencies of the limbs may vary from complete absence (amelia) to partial absence (phocomelia). Every gradation may occur and only one limb or all four limbs may be affected, or even absent.

There may be absence of one or more bones on the medial and lateral aspects of the arm or leg and this may lead to deformities such as a Madelung's deformity (radial deviation of both hands) due to a short or absent radius or varus of both feet due to absent tibia. Often the digits on the side of the absent long bone are also deficient or absent.

The cause of limb differences is usually drugs such as thalidomide in the first trimester of pregnancy. Other causes include irradiation, rubella, true genetic abnormalities or unknown aetiological factors.

Macromelia and macrodactyly

Overgrowth of the limb may also occur. It may be due to a true genetic abnormality when individual digits may have overgrown (usually three digits), or may involve the whole limb. In the latter case, congenital lymphangiectasis may be responsible.

Upper Limb Conditions

Drugs and irradiation

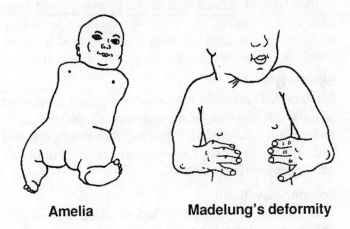

Amelia

Madelung's deformity

Idiopathic conditions

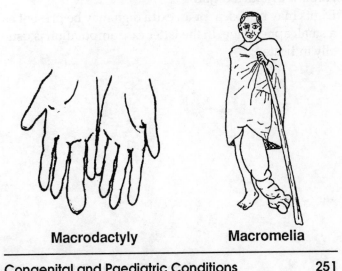

Macrodactyly

Macromelia

Trigger thumb and little finger

A contracture of the fibrous flexor sheath of the thumb or little finger may occur. This is usually symmetrical and affects either both thumbs or both little fingers. The digits may be held in fixed flexion or they may permit 'triggering' or 'snapping' into extension due to a secondary nodule on the tendon suddenly being released from the constricted flexor sheath like a tight cork in a bottle.

Syndactyly

Syndactyly is fusion of one or more digits. It may affect all the digits together, or, more commonly, pairs of digits such as index and middle finger together or with the ring and little finger fused. The limbs are usually, but not always, symmetrically affected.

Lobster claw hand

This is different in that there is lack of fusion with usually only two digits creating a claw-like deformity as illustrated.

Absent or extra digits

Digits may be absent or an extra digit may be present as a small appendage. In the latter case amputation is usually indicated.

Upper Limb Conditions

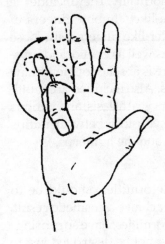

Trigger finger

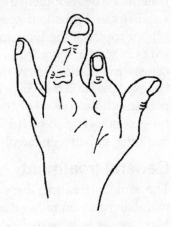

Syndactyly

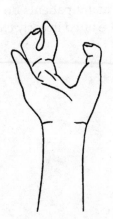

Lobster claw hand

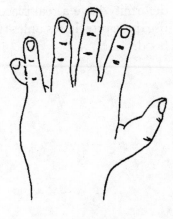

Extra digit

Other developmental upper limb deformities

These are discussed elsewhere and may be part of a generalised developmental abnormality. They include the short upper limbs and spade-like 'chubby' fingers in achondroplasia, the long spider-like fingers with loose joints in Marfan's syndrome, as well as craniocleidodys-ostosis, a condition where there is absence of membrane bones of the skull and clavicles. Also included are multiple osteochondromata of diaphyseal aclasis, and various types of bony fusion such as a synostosis between radius and ulna, or between the ulna and the humerus.

General treatment

The aim, in treating these deformities, should be to maintain function rather than achieve a cosmetic result. Many patients, despite the deformities, have surprisingly good function and this must not be destroyed just to improve the appearance.

Artificial limbs specially tailored to the individual deformity have a real place, but many patients do not use these prostheses unless they are fitted in early childhood.

Treatment

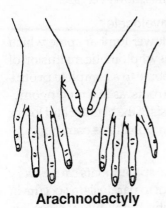

Arachnodactyly

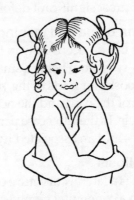

Craniocleidodysostosis

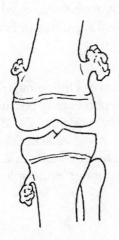

X-ray appearance
of multiple
osteochondromata

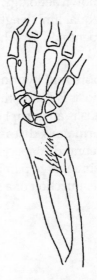

X-ray appearance of
radio-ulnar synostosis

Spinal Conditions

These are discussed in more detail in Chapter 11. The four most significant deformities, however, are:

Spina bifida and meningomyelocele

This is a defect usually in the lower lumbar spine which may vary from being a small asymptomatic malfusion of the posterior parts of the vertebrae to a complete protrusion of the cord and the nerve roots, as in a meningomyelocele. In the latter case paralysis of the bladder and lower limbs and an associated hydrocephalus is common.

Scoliosis

This is a lateral curvature of the spine and its causes vary from a congenital hemivertebra to paralysis, as occurs in conditions such as poliomyelitis, but in many cases it is of unknown aetiology.

Unequal limb lengths will produce a scoliosis which is compensated for when the patient sits down or bends forward.

Kyphosis and kyphos

A kyphosis is a smooth forward curve of the spine, while a kyphos is an abrupt curve. A kyphosis may be due to Scheuermann's disease (an osteochondritis of the intervertebral disc spaces which mainly affects the thoracic vertebrae) or to paralysis. A kyphos is usually due to a fracture, infection or a secondary tumour of the spine.

A Simple Guide to Orthopaedics

Spinal Conditions

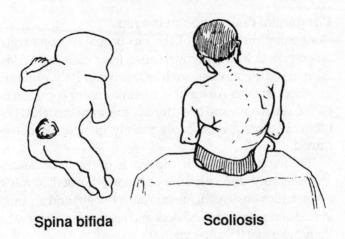

Spina bifida

Scoliosis

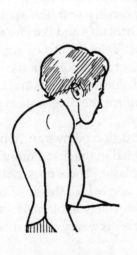

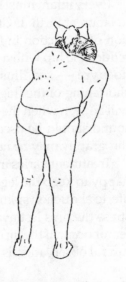

Kyphosis

Kyphoscoliosis

Lower Limb Conditions

Hip conditions

Congenital dislocation of the hip

Congenital dislocation of the hip probably has a combined genetic and hormonal cause. It is much more common in some countries, such as Japan and Italy, and rare in others such as Africa. It is six times more common in girls than in boys and one–third of cases are bilateral. The bilateral cases are probably mainly genetically determined.

The main defects which appear in untreated cases are an upwardly dislocated hip, a poorly formed, sloping acetabulum (instead of the normal 60° shelf) and an anteverted and poorly formed neck and head of femur (greater than the usual 35° anteversion).

Every infant must be examined for dislocation or subluxation at birth. If CDH is present there will be limitation of abduction in flexion, usually with the ability to reduce the hip with a click (Ortolani's and Barlow's manoeuvre — see illustration). Telescoping of the hip, shortening of the thigh and increased folds in the thigh will be seen when the hip is dislocated. X-rays and ultrasound should be used to confirm the diagnosis and arthrography may be necessary.

Treatment varies from abduction pillows and a bulky nappy to keep the legs abducted in the first 3 months of life, to abduction splints and plaster. These must not over stress the hips lest avascular necrosis of the head of the femur occur. If the hips are completely stable at 6 months, careful observation is all that is necessary in most cases.

Lower Limb Conditions

Congenital dislocation of the hip

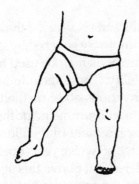

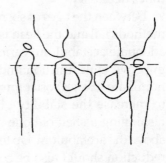

Asymmetrical skin folds

X-ray appearance of CDH

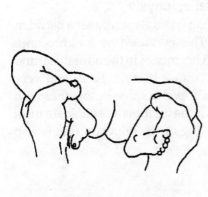

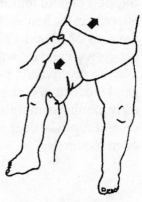

**Limited hip abduction
— Ortolani's test**

Hip telescoping

In many cases, however, an infolding 'limbus' of capsule prevents concentric reduction, necessitating open reduction if splinting fails. A persistent anteversion of the head and neck of the femur may require external rotation osteotomy of the upper femur with plate fixation. Open reduction of the hip and excision of the limbus is sometimes necessary.

Between the ages of six months and six years, if these methods fail and the head is incompletely covered by an adequate acetabulum, various methods may be used to improve joint function and stability. These include innominate (Salter) osteotomy, or various other methods to increase the stability of the acetabulum including fashioning a shelf of bone or displacement of the ilium above the acetabulum. Up to the age of twelve years open reduction should also be considered but above this age the alternatives are no treatment, an osteotomy of the upper femur to give stability (Schantz) or in adult life a cementless total hip replacement.

Slipped capital femoral epiphysis

Slipping of the femoral epiphysis is usually seen between the ages of 10 and 15. This is caused by an imbalance between sex and growth hormones in the adolescent and may be precipitated by minor trauma. Early and very gentle reduction of the slipped epiphysis, together with early pinning of the hip, is the treatment of choice in most cases. Prophylactic pinning of the opposite side is also often required.

Lower Limb Conditions

Congenital dislocation of the hip

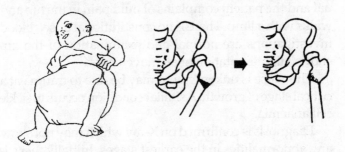

Abduction pillow

Schantz osteotomy

Slipped epiphysis

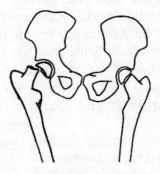

**X-ray appearance of a
slipped epiphysis**

Perthes' disease

Perthes' disease is an osteochondritis of the femoral capital epiphysis and is due to disturbance of the blood supply to the femoral head. Children usually present between the ages of 5 and 10. The onset tends to be gradual and the patient complains of mild pain in the hip and walks with a limp. There is no constitutional upset, blood investigations are normal and examination of the hip shows slight limitation of all movements.

The cause is unknown but may be due to trauma at a critical stage of growth. A similar condition occurs in sickle cell anaemia.

Diagnosis is confirmed on X-ray which may not show any abnormalities in the earliest stages. Initially there is flattening and decrease in the depth of the epiphysis which becomes denser and fragmented. Nuclear scanning will show deficient uptake in the ossific nucleus of the head.

The head gradually revascularises over a period of two years but the head and neck usually remain permanently flattened and deformed in severe cases.

Treatment should aim to contain the softened femoral head in the acetabulum and prevent full weight-bearing in the early stages. Initially the child should be admitted to hospital and treated with skin traction in abduction. As soon as the pain has settled this is replaced by an abduction walking frame with gradually increasing weight-bearing.

Severe cases are later complicated by osteoarthritis and may require total hip replacement.

Transient synovitis

A transient synovitis of the hip is not uncommon in the first 10 years of life. The patient complains of severe hip

Lower Limb Conditions

Perthes' Disease

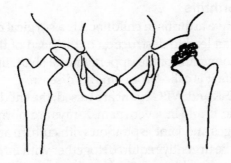

**X-ray appearance of
unilateral Perthes' disease**

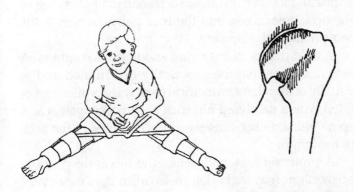

Abduction splint

**X-ray appearance of
old Perthes' disease**

pain with the hip flexed, initially abducted then adducted and *externally* rotated. X-rays and white cell count are initially normal with a normal or slightly raised ESR. The patient should be treated with Russell traction and bed rest as the differential diagnosis is a low grade infection such as tuberculosis or Perthes' disease.

Septic arthritis

An infective arthritis in childhood is a surgical emergency as it can lead to destruction of the head of the femur and osteomyelitis of the upper femoral shaft. In the first year of life it is called Tom Smith's disease.

The ESR and WBC count are raised, the child is usually pyrexic, ill and in severe pain. X-rays are normal in the early stages and joint aspiration with culture and drainage may be urgently required, together with intravenous antibiotics after blood for culture has been taken.

Coxa vara and valga and protrusio acetabuli

Coxa vara and valga refer to a decrease and increase respectively in the angle between the head and neck of the femur and its shaft. Protrusio acetabuli is an extension of the acetabular fossa into the true pelvis, which limits movement at the hip joint.

A mild degree of coxa vara and valga is common. A severe degree may be genetically determined and is usually bilateral. Asymmetrical coxa valga is often associated with a paralysed hip such as in poliomyelitis and spina bifida. Other causes include fractures of the neck of the femur.

A protrusio acetabuli, when the hip is deep in the acetabulum, may lead to later osteoarthritis, as may a very shallow acetabulum.

Hip Conditions

Transient synovitis

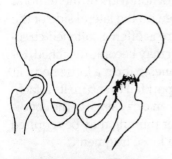

Flexed, externally rotated and abducted

Infective arthritis

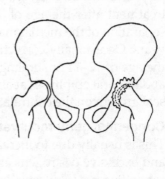

X-ray appearance of the destruction of the acetabulum and femoral head

Coxa vara

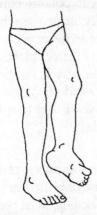

X-ray appearance of osteoarthritis

Coxa valga

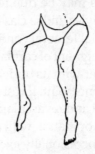

Associated with paralysis

Knee conditions

Genu varum and genu valgum

Knock knees and bow legs are common in childhood and are often familial. If unassociated with poliomyelitis, injury or bone disease, they usually improve without treatment after the age of 3. The maximum acceptable separation of the medial malleoli is 7.5cm (3 inches) at 3 years. Occasionally corrective osteotomy is required at the age of 12–14 or stapling epiphysiodesis of the tibial and femoral epiphyses at about 10 years to stop epiphyseal growth on the contralateral side.

Congenital genu recurvatum

This is usually due to increased intra-amniotic pressure and excessive oestrogens at the time of birth. Immobilisation in a *padded* plaster, in as much flexion as possible for three weeks will usually effect a cure. Occasionally this condition is associated with arthrogryposis or with fibrotic and tight quadriceps and these conditions are difficult to treat and will usually require operation.

Osteochondritis

A painful knee, particularly between the ages of 10–15 years may be due to an osteochondritis of the femoral condyles and is classically seen on the lateral side of the medial femoral condyle. There is often a softened circular segment of cartilage which may become detached, together with its underlying bone, to form a loose body in the knee joint. If rest and support fail to secure its attachment and revascularisation at an early stage of the condition, operation with drilling or pinning may be required and occasionally excision of a loose fragment.

Knee Conditions

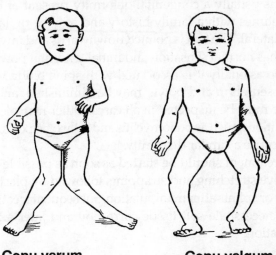

Genu varum ('bow legs')

Genu valgum ('knock knees')

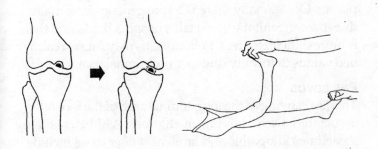

X-ray appearance of osteochondritis

Genu recurvatum

Ankle and foot conditions

Talipes equino varus

This is usually a congenital deformity present at birth, sometimes with a family history and may be unilateral or bilateral. The foot is pointed downwards and inwards, and has normal sensation and initially normal power.

Occasionally it is associated with spina bifida when both sensation and power may be diminished, and the spine must be inspected in all cases. Other neurological conditions, such as poliomyelitis and arthrogryposis, may also cause a similar deformity.

Treatment should be started as soon as possible with passive stretching and strapping, followed by plaster of Paris or splints after manipulation. Subsequent treatment may necessitate soft tissue correction and later a bony operation.

Talipes calcaneo valgus

This is the opposite deformity to equino varus and the foot is dorsiflexed and everted. It is usually caused by intrauterine pressure on the foetus and most cases are easily corrected by passive stretching, strapping and plaster. Occasionally there is a true genetic abnormality due to a congenital vertical talus or spina bifida and this is more difficult to treat. Poliomyelitis may cause a calcaneo valgus deformity due to muscle imbalance.

Pes cavus

This is a clawing of the longitudinal arch of the foot often associated with clawing of the toes. Mild cases are sometimes idiopathic and familial. Other cases include neurological conditions such as spina bifida, peroneal muscular atrophy, Friedreich's ataxia and poliomyelitis, as may vascular insufficiency.

Ankle and Foot Conditions

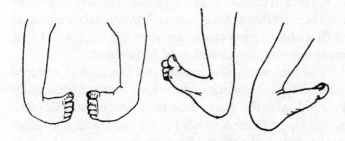

Talipes equino varus

Talipes calcaneo valgus

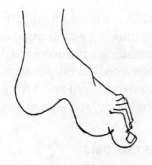

Pes cavus ('claw foot')

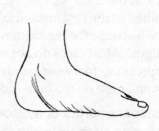

Pes planus ('flat foot')

In severe cases callosities may develop under the forefoot and toes and may necessitate special footwear and occasionally soft tissue or bony correction.

Pes planus

Flat feet is a common condition with the medial border of the foot in contact with the ground and the foot everted. There is often a family history. It may also be associated with a short tendo calcaneus with the valgus flat foot compensating for limitation of dorsiflexion.

The foot is usually mobile and the arch is restored when the patient stands on the toes. It may occasionally be rigid, and the cause may be a congenital calcaneonavicular or other subtaloid bony bar leading to peroneal spasm and a spastic flat foot.

Mobile flat feet seldom require treatment except for an occasional small raise on the inner side of the heel or an arch support. Spastic flat feet sometimes require a subtaloid arthrodesis.

Metatarsus adductus

This is a congenital deformity with the forefoot adducted and the child walking with an intoeing gait. It may be limited to the first metatarsal (metatarsus primus varus) in which case the big toe may be pivoted laterally (hallux valgus). Most cases do not require treatment apart from appropriate footwear, passive stretching, and sometimes a small raise on the outer side of the shoe.

Osteochondritis or avascular necrosis

This may affect the navicular (Köhler's disease) or head of the second metatarsal (Freiberg's disease) and both are probably due to trauma, with interruption of the blood supply resulting in avascular changes. Gradual revascularisation, with residual deformity and little disability

Ankle and Foot Conditions

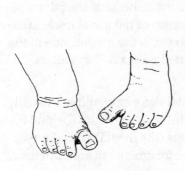

Metatarsus adductus

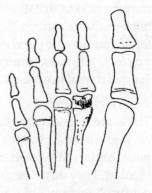

X-ray appearance of Freiberg's disease — osteochondritis of second metatarsal head

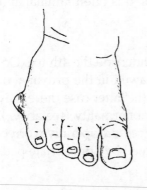

Exostosis of fifth metatarsal head

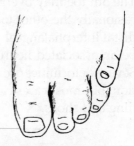

Syndactyly and overriding fifth toe

usually occurs with conservative treatment with rest and perhaps supports.

Exostoses

These are often associated with an overlying bursa and may be due to irritation by footwear. They include the back of the calcaneus, the base or head of the 5th metatarsal (bunionette), and dorsum of the metatarsals in cavus feet. The most common site is the medial side of the 1st metatarsal head associated with a hallux valgus.

Accessory bones

These are due to a congenital deformity and are usually asymptomatic. They include the os trigonum (behind the talus) and os tibialis externus (the medial side of the navicular). They do not require treatment but are sometimes confused with an old fracture.

Syndactyly

This may be variable in extent and implies partial fusion of the web of one or more toes. It is often familial and seldom requires treatment.

Other toe deformities

The 5th toe may override or underride the 4th toe. Occasionally the other toes are clawed in the proximal or distal interphalangeal joint. In the latter case there may be an associated neurological abnormality (see above). Severe deformities occasionally require operative correction, but most cases can be treated by appropriate padding and shoes.

Chapter 8

Musculoskeletal Neoplasms

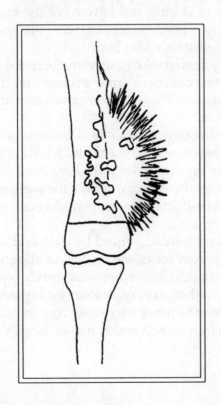

Introduction

Musculoskeletal tumours can be divided into:

1. Primary bone tumours
2. Secondary deposits in bone
3. Soft tissue tumours

Primary tumours in bone can be divided, in turn, into benign or those which are localised and will not spread to other parts of the body, and malignant or those which may metastasise or spread elsewhere and cause death. The benign tumours can be subdivided into those which were present at birth and have a genetic link such as multiple osteochondromata and those apparently occurring for the first time after birth.

Primary tumours also have been subdivided into those arising from bone, those from cartilage and those from the bone marrow. There is sometimes an overlap between these origins.

Bone tumours can also be classified according to whether they arise from the medulla (Ewing's sarcoma or multiple myeloma), from the bone itself (osteogenic sarcoma, chondrosarcoma) or from the overlying periosteum (non-ossifying fibroma, periosteal osteogenic sarcoma).

Secondary tumours spread by the blood stream are commonly from breast (nearly half of all secondaries), thyroid, bronchus, kidney, prostate, cervix, ovary, colon or bone but other primary tumours may spread to bone.

Soft tissue tumours may arise from muscle, fibrous tissue, synovia, lymph nodes, nerves, blood vessels, fat and skin.

Diagnosis

The diagnosis of bone tumours is made on clinical and radiological grounds, with other investigations including bone scanning and blood analysis. A benign tumour is usually painless, static in size, with a well-defined edge on X-ray, and 'cold' on bone scanning in the adult. Blood investigations are usually negative. A malignant tumour may be in a classical site, growing rapidly and be hot and painful. It may have classical X-ray appearance such as 'Codman's triangles' and 'sunray spicules' with indistinct margins. It may also infiltrate the soft tissues and be 'hot' on bone scans.

Blood investigations may show a raised alkaline phosphatase, an abnormal electrophoretic curve for plasma proteins and possibly other abnormalities.

In secondary bone tumours a known primary site, and the typical appearance of multiple secondaries often helps to make the diagnosis. Trephine or fine needle biopsy may still be necessary for confirmation.

In tumours such as multiple myeloma and other haematological malignancies, additional investigations including a bone marrow biopsy, and sometimes urine analysis for Bence–Jones proteins may be needed.

A final diagnosis may have to rely on a biopsy which is essential in all suspected primary malignant bone tumours.

Benign Neoplasms Classification

Cartilage
Enchondroma
Ecchondroma
Chondroblastoma
Osteochondroma

Bone
Bone cysts — uniloculated
multiloculated
Osteoma
Osteoid osteoma
Osteoblastoma

Soft tissue

Fibrous tissue
Fibrous dysplasia
Non-ossifying fibroma
Fibrous cortical defect
Neurofibroma

Vascular
Eosinophilic granuloma
Aneurysmal bone cyst
Giant cell tumour 'benign'
Haemangioma

Benign Neoplasms

Common sites of occurrence

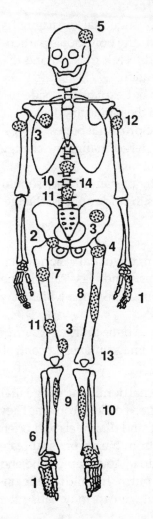

1. Enchondroma and ecchondroma

2. Chondroblastoma

3. Osteochondroma

4. Bone cysts

5. Osteoma

6. Osteoid osteoma

7. Osteoblastoma

8. Fibrous dysplasia

9. Non-ossifying fibroma and fibrocortical defect

10. Neurofibroma

11. Eosinophilic granuloma

12. Aneurysmal bone cysts

13. Giant cell tumours

14. Haemangioma

Benign Cartilaginous Neoplasms

Enchondroma and ecchondroma

An enchondroma is a benign, congenital cartilaginous tumour which may be present in any bone but is particularly common in the hands and feet. It may expand the bone and have flecks of calcification.

An ecchondroma is similar but expands outside the bone and is mainly confined to the hands and feet.

Enchondromata in the more proximal bones, and especially in the pelvis, may undergo malignant change and develop into chondrosarcomata.

If these tumours are growing or painful they should be excised. If there is any suggestion of neoplastic change, biopsy is essential.

Chondroblastoma

A chondroblastoma is a benign, congenital lesion which is usually present in an epiphysis and classically in the femoral head. It is a small circumscribed area which may have flecks of calcification.

The treatment is curettage and bone grafting if symptomatic, often performed under image intensifier control.

Osteochondroma

Diaphyseal aclasis is an autosomal dominant, congenital lesion which produces multiple osteochondromata. They arise from the epiphyseal plate and diaphysis and often have a stalk protruding *away* from the epiphyseal plate with a cauliflower-shaped cartilaginous cap on the end which may have an overlying bursa. In children the unossified radiotranslucent cartilage cap may cause the

Benign Neoplasms

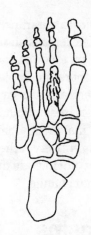 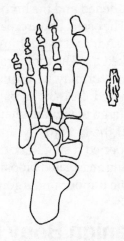

X-ray appearance of an enchondroma and ecchondroma

Treatment: excision if malignant or symptomatic — otherwise conservative

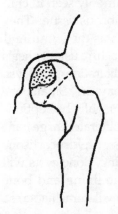 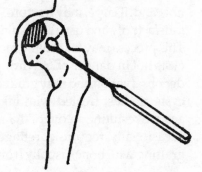

X-ray appearance of a chondroblastoma

Treatment: curettage and bone graft

tumour to look smaller on X-ray than it actually is. Growth disturbances are common at the epiphysis which may be broadened and the limb shortened.

The osteochondroma has a classical appearance on X-ray and, as it is often multiple, other lesions should be looked for. The tumours may press on tendons and ligaments, or may be prominent and therefore liable to be knocked. In 1–3% of patients the cartilaginous cap may undergo malignant change to a chondrosarcoma.

If the lesion is symptomatic or malignant change is suspected it should be excised in its entirety rather than taking an isolated biopsy which may not include the part of the tumour undergoing malignant change.

Benign Bony Neoplasms

Bone cysts

Bone cysts are congenital, benign, unilocular or multilocular defects in the bone and are commonly seen in children. They usually have a lining of fibrous tissue. They commonly occur in long bones such as the femur and tibia and, if large, may fracture. The fracture usually heals satisfactorily and usually results in obliteration of the cyst. This process may take many months or years. Small bone cysts not in danger of fracturing can usually be kept under observation and may gradually obliterate. Large bone cysts are best treated with injections of hydrocortisone acetate resulting in over 80% resolving. Bone cysts will occasionally require curettage of the lining and bone grafting with bone, usually from the ipsilateral iliac crest.

Benign Neoplasms

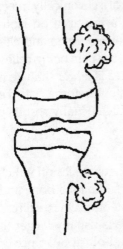

**X-ray appearance of
an osteochondroma**

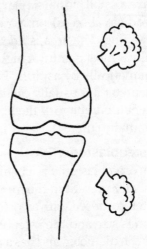

**Treatment: excision
if symptomatic**

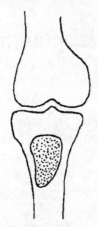

**X-ray appearance
of a bone cyst**

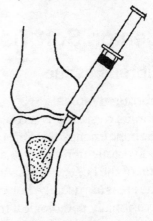

**Treatment:
hydrocortisone injection
or excise and bone graft**

Osteoid osteoma

An osteoid osteoma is a cystic area in a bone which may have a small nidus (similar to that of a chronically infected Brodie's abscess) on X-ray and a hot area on isotope scanning. The area is lined by fibrous tissue and classically is most painful at night, with the pain being relieved dramatically by aspirin. If the area is larger than 2cm in diameter it is usually called an osteoblastoma. The treatment is curettage of the lesion which usually results in a dramatic cure.

Osteoblastoma

An osteoblastoma is a benign, congenital lesion which is usually present in the metaphysis of a long bone and is often confused with an osteoid osteoma. One differentiation is size and the osteoblastoma is usually larger than 2cm in diameter, and has a punched-out appearance with a clearly demarcated margin. The treatment is curettage and bone grafting if large.

Benign Soft Tissue Neoplasms

Fibrous tissue

Fibrous dysplasia

Fibrous dysplasia is a congenital defect and may affect one bone (monostotic fibrous dysplasia) or more than one (polyostotic fibrous dysplasia). X-rays show an expansion of the bone, cystic spaces and increased trabeculae. The areas are usually 'hot' on isotope bone scanning and occasionally pathological fractures may occur.

If the areas are large, or pathological fractures occur, they may require curettage, bone grafting and occasionally internal fixation.

Benign Neoplasms

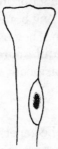

X-ray appearance of an osteoid osteoma

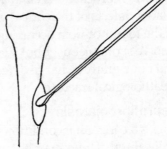

Treatment: curettage and biopsy

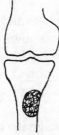

X-ray appearance of an osteoblastoma

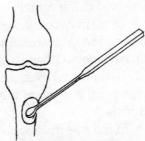

Treatment: curettage and bone graft

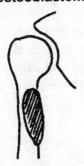

X-ray appearance of fibrous dysplasia

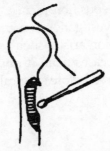

Treatment: curettage and bone graft if in danger of fracture

Musculoskeletal Neoplasms

Non-ossifying fibroma

A fibrous cortical defect and a non-ossifying fibroma are related defects of the cortex, usually of a long bone such as the femur or tibia occurring in children. They usually resolve spontaneously, but if large, may require curettage and bone grafting. Large defects may occasionally cause a pathological fracture.

Neurofibromatosis

This is a congenital condition which may be generalised or localised. There may be multiple neurofibromata affecting the spinal, cranial or peripheral nerves. If large these may lead to paralysis, chiefly through pressure on the cord in the spinal canal.

There may be cutaneous neurofibromata and characteristic brown discolouration of the skin known as 'cafe au lait' spots. Other associated features may include scoliosis, limb weakness, overgrowth of a limb or fractures due to infiltration of the mid tibia causing a pseudoarthrosis.

In the rare instance of malignant change the neurofibroma starts growing and becomes a fibrosarcoma. Occasionally the sarcomatous change may also occur in the cutaneous fibromata.

Investigation is usually only necessary when a complication arises, such as pressure on the spinal cord. In these cases plain X-ray, CT scanning and MRI may be required before surgical excision of the neurofibroma.

Benign Neoplasms

Non-ossifying fibroma

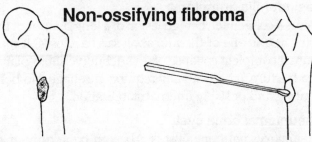

**X-ray appearance of a
non-ossifying fibroma**

**Treatment: curettage
and bone graft if
complications likely**

Neurofibromatosis

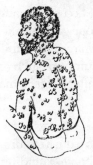

Multiple neurofibromata

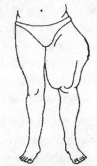

Limb overgrowth

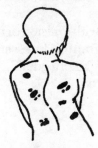

Scoliosis

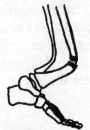

**X-ray appearance of a mid-
tibial pseudoarthrosis**

Vascular

Eosinophilic granuloma

This is a congenital, benign lesion of a long bone or of the spine and is one of the mucopolysaccharidoses. It may cause a complete collapse of a vertebra (vertebra plana) or a fracture. It occasionally requires curettage and bone grafting and possibly internal stabilisation.

Aneurysmal bone cyst

An aneurysmal bone cyst is a benign bone tumour of young adults, usually involving the shaft of a long bone but may also affect a vertebra. There is often expansion of the bone which is filled with blood. The bone is weakened and may fracture.

The cyst should be curetted, if accessible, and filled with bone graft if necessary. The bone graft is taken from the ipsilateral iliac crest. Fractures may need stabilisation with plates or nails. Inaccessible tumours such as those involving the spine, or recurrences after surgery, may need low dosage radiotherapy.

'Benign' giant cell tumour

This may present in every gradation from a circumscribed tumour at the *epiphysis* of a long bone extending to the articular margin, to a highly malignant tumour (described below) extending into the soft tissues.

Benign tumours are best treated with excision of non-essential bones or curettage and grafting in essential bones. Liquid nitrogen into the cavity before grafting will diminish the likelihood of recurrence.

Benign Neoplasms

Eosinophilic granuloma

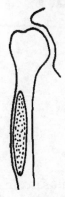 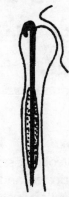

X-ray appearance of an eosinophilic granuloma

Treatment: internal stabilisation after curettage

Benign giant cell tumour

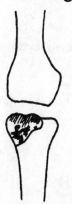 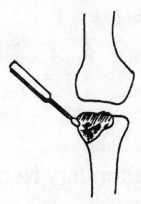

X-ray appearance of a circumscribed giant cell tumour

Treatment: curettage and bone graft

Malignant Neoplasms Classification

Primary Neoplasms

Cartilage

Chondrosarcoma

Bone

Cortex

Osteogenic sarcoma
Periosteal and parosteal osteogenic sarcoma
Paget's osteogenic sarcoma

Medulla

Malignant giant cell tumour
Ewing's sarcoma
Multiple myeloma

Soft tissue

Fibrosarcoma and malignant fibrohistiocytoma
Rhabdomyosarcoma
Synoviosarcoma
Basal squamous cell carcinoma and malignant
melanoma
Lipoma
Angiosarcoma

Secondary Neoplasms

Malignant Neoplasms

Common sites of occurrence

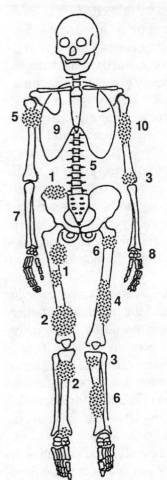

1. Chondrosarcoma

2. Osteogenic sarcoma

3. Giant cell tumour

4. Ewing's sarcoma

5. Multiple myeloma

6. Malignant fibrohistiocytoma

7. Rhabdomyosarcoma

8. Synoviosarcoma

9. Liposarcoma

10. Angiosarcoma

Malignant Cartilaginous Neoplasms

Chondrosarcoma

Chondrosarcoma can be primary or secondary to an osteochondroma, enchondroma or ecchondroma. They usually occur in the shafts of long bones, the pelvis or the scapula, but may occasionally occur in the hands and feet where they are usually secondary to an enchondroma.

Diagnosis is made by clinical history which may include a previous benign tumour plus a gradually increasing bony mass which is usually tender and warm. X-rays show a tumour, usually with expansion of the bone, indefinite edges with or without specks of calcification. Bone scanning will show an area of increased uptake. Confirmation of the diagnosis requires biopsy. Histology will show cartilage cells with mitotic figures. In slow growing tumours the clinical history of increased growth may be necessary to confirm the histological diagnosis.

A chondrosarcoma is usually much slower growing than an osteogenic sarcoma and the prognosis is better.

The treatment of a tumour secondary to an osteochondroma is complete local excision. At least 3 cm of normal bone should be excised on each side of the lesion if possible. In other tumours resection of bone at least 6 cm clear of the tumour should be aimed for, including the joint itself if necessary. If complete excision is not possible then amputation should be carried out.

Most tumours are radioresistant. Local palliative resection of isolated pulmonary secondary deposits is often indicated.

Malignant Neoplasms

Chondrosarcoma

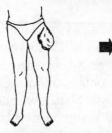
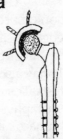

Primary chondrosarcoma of upper femur

Treatment: excision, ceramic and titanium hip and femur

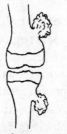
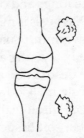

Chondrosarcoma; secondary to diaphyseal aclasis

Treatment: complete excision

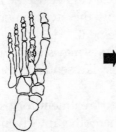
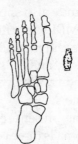

Chondrosarcoma; secondary to enchondroma

Treatment: excision

Malignant Bone Neoplasms

Cortex

Osteogenic sarcoma

An osteogenic sarcoma is a highly malignant tumour occurring most commonly in the 15–25 year old age group. It may also occur in Paget's disease in old age and as a parosteal osteogenic sarcoma in middle age.

The metaphysis of the upper tibia, lower femur and upper humerus are the most common sites but it may occur at other sites. There is a variable degree of bone, cartilage and fibrous tissue found on pathological examination, and the tumour metastasises via the blood stream to the lungs and other organs.

Diagnosis is made by the history of the pain, swelling and warmth, usually in the metaphyseal region of a long bone in a young adult. X-rays show variable degrees of bone destruction and regeneration with elevation of the periosteum (Codman's triangles) and perforation of the tumour through the periosteum (sunray spicules). There is often soft tissue infiltration and no clear definition of the margins of the tumour.

Isotope bone scan will usually show a very 'hot' area and may also show 'skip' areas higher up the bone. CT and MRI scans may also show the involvement of soft tissue and medullary involvement.

X-ray and CT scan of the lungs may show evidence of secondary involvement. Biopsy is essential to confirm the diagnosis.

The present recommended treatment for osteogenic sarcoma is three courses of chemotherapy given at about 3-weekly intervals, followed by amputation at least 6 cm above the highest level of tumour. The chemotherapy is

Malignant Neoplasms

Osteogenic Sarcoma

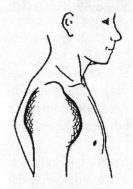

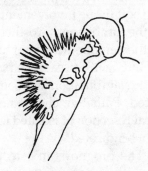

Osteogenic sarcoma

X-ray appearance of an osteogenic sarcoma showing sun-ray spicules and Codman's triangle

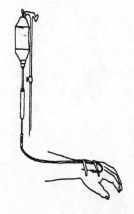

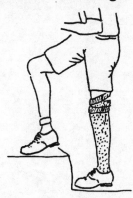

Treatment: chemotherapy, followed by amputation, occasionally local excision and bone replacement may be required

then continued for 1–2 more years. At the time of amputation the response of the tumour to the preoperative chemotherapy is assessed and this is changed if necessary.

In the case of low-grade osteogenic sarcoma and parosteal osteogenic sarcoma without significant overlying soft tissue involvement, there is a place for resection of the tumour and prosthetic replacement or arthrodesis of the neighbouring joint followed by chemotherapy.

In Paget's disease the prognosis is very poor, but palliative amputation and sometimes radiotherapy is indicated. Palliative chemotherapy and radiotherapy and local resection of isolated lung secondaries is also sometimes indicated.

The prognosis in osteogenic sarcoma has been improved with chemotherapy but still has only a 30–50% survival rate compared with 5–20% before chemotherapy.

Malignant Neoplasms

Osteogenic Sarcoma

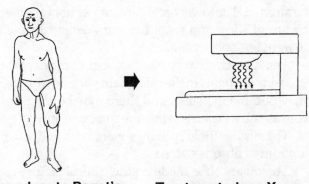

Secondary to Paget's disease

Treatment: deep X-ray therapy and palliative amputation

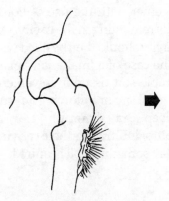

X-ray appearance of a parosteal sarcoma of the upper femur

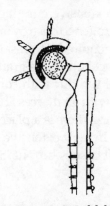

Treatment: total hip and upper femoral replacement

Medulla

Giant cell tumour

A giant cell tumour may present as any grade from benign to malignant. It usually involves the epiphysis of a long bone but occasionally other bones such as the pelvis may be affected. The lower femur and upper tibia are the most common sites, and most tumours extend to the joint margin but not beyond.

The tumour usually has clear-cut margins and often expands the bone. In the malignant varieties the margins may become indistinct and there may be fractures and considerable expansion into the surrounding soft tissues.

The histopathology shows giant cells and a variable amount of fibrous stroma.

The diagnosis is made on the clinical picture as well as the X-ray appearance which shows an expanded cortex with no new trabeculae. Bone scans usually show a 'cold' tumour with surrounding hyperaemia.

Treatment should be excision if possible. Alternatively extensive curettage, together with the use of liquid nitrogen to destroy any cells remaining in the cavity, will be required. The residual cavity should then be filled with cancellous bone graft. In the case of a 'malignant' giant cell tumour with considerable soft tissue involvement, or with an inaccessible surgical site or following a recurrence, there is a place for deep X-ray therapy.

In very extensive tumours, infiltrating the overlying soft tissues, amputation may sometimes be required.

Malignant Neoplasms

Giant Cell Tumour

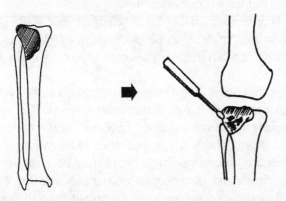

X-ray appearance of a 'benign' giant cell tumour: extends to articular surface with well defined margin

Treatment: curettage, liquid nitrogen and bone graft; complete excision if possible

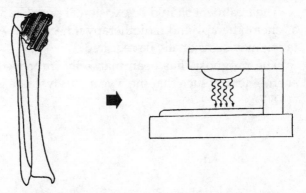

X-ray appearance of a malignant giant cell tumour: poorly defined margins

Treatment: deep X-ray therapy or amputation

Ewing's sarcoma

Ewing's sarcoma occurs commonly in children and occasionally in older age groups. It classically involves the shaft of a long bone, especially the femur, tibia and humerus, but may occur elsewhere.

It is a tumour arising from lymphocytes in the bone marrow and may resemble secondaries from a neuroblastoma. It often metastasises early and may grow rapidly.

The diagnosis is made by a history of a hot swelling which is tender and may mimic osteomyelitis. There may be rapid growth with a raised ESR and white cell count.

Classically the X-ray appearance is elevation of the periosteum, 'onion peeling'. There may be 'sun-ray spicules' similar to an osteogenic sarcoma but the lesion usually extends more into the diaphysis than the metaphysis. Bone scanning will show 'hot' areas. Biopsy is essential and often shows 'pseudopus' which is sterile and shows lymphocytes and no organisms on microscopy.

The treatment should be excision, if possible, as well as chemotherapy and radiotherapy if necessary. Amputation may occasionally be required.

The prognosis has been markedly improved with chemotherapy such that the 5 year survival rate is now 70–80%.

Malignant Neoplasms

Ewing's Sarcoma

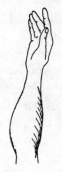

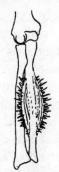

Ewing's sarcoma

X-ray appearance of a
Ewing's sarcoma
showing onion peeling
and spicules

Treatment

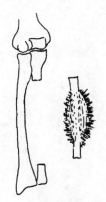

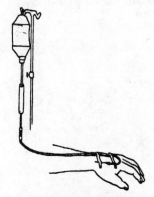

Excision

Chemotherapy or
radiotherapy

Myeloma

(Solitary and multiple myeloma)

This is a tumour of the bone marrow in adults with considerable numbers of plasma cells present on biopsy. It may be solitary but most cases are multiple with deposits in the skull, vertebrae and other bones.

The diagnosis is made on a general systemic upset accompanied by multiple tender areas and sometimes pathological fractures. There may also be severe back pain due to spinal secondaries and sometimes paraplegia.

Radiological diagnosis depends on the presence of classic 'punched-out' areas in bone plus a bone marrow biopsy or tumour showing the characteristic plasma cells. The serum proteins usually show a reversed albumin/globulin ratio on electrophoresis. The urine in 40% of cases shows Bence–Jones protein (proteins which cause cloudiness on heating that disappear on boiling).

The treatment is chemotherapy and radiotherapy if necessary. Pathological fractures will usually require internal stabilisation but the bone may be extremely vascular and bleed profusely.

Malignant Neoplasms

Multiple Myeloma

X-ray appearance

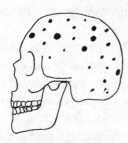

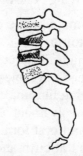

**Skull showing
'punched-out' areas**

**Spine: collapsed
vertebrae with
normal discs**

Treatment

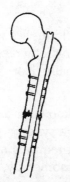

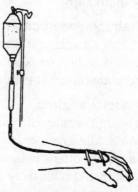

**Internal fixation of
pathological fractures**

**Chemotherapy and
radiotherapy**

Malignant Soft Tissue Neoplasms

Soft tissue tumours may involve only the soft tissues themselves or may be adherent to or even erode into the underlying bone or joint.

Fibroma, fibrous dysplasia and malignant fibrohistiocytoma

A benign fibroma radiologically appears as a cleanly punched-out bone defect (fibrous cortical defect or non-ossifying fibroma). Fibrous dysplasia may show extensive involvement of one or more long bones with expansion and cyst formation and possible fractures. This is present at birth and is called monostotic (one bone) or polyostotic (more than one bone) fibrous dysplasia.

Malignant fibrohistiocytoma may involve any bone or the fibrous tissue overlying bone. Radical excision, including the involved bone, is usually possible with replacement, otherwise amputation may be necessary. Occasionally the tumours will respond to radiotherapy or chemotherapy.

Rhabdomyosarcoma

This is a malignant tumour of skeletal muscles which requires radical excision. It responds to radiotherapy and chemotherapy, but the prognosis is usually poor.

Synoviosarcoma

A benign tumour of synovial tissue is known as a synovioma. Malignant change is known as a synovio-sarcoma which often metastasises early. It requires radical excision and often deep X-ray and chemotherapy.

Malignant Neoplasms

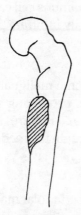

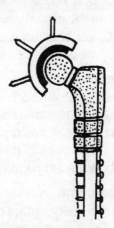

X-ray appearance of a fibrohistiocytoma of proximal femur

Treatment: excision followed by hip and femoral replacement

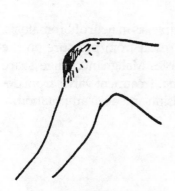

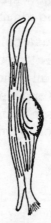

Synoviosarcoma

Rhabdomyosarcoma of biceps brachii

Basal and squamous cell carcinomata

Basal cell carcinoma (BCC) of the skin seldom metastasizes but may erode locally, eventually infiltrating and destroying the underlying bone. Squamous cell carcinoma (SCC) and melanoma may not only infiltrate the underlying structures but may metastasise.

Liposarcoma

These are common and seldom become malignant. Occasionally malignant change occurs producing a liposarcoma which shows rapid growth and requires radical excision. Occasionally these may occur in the medulla of a long bone and expand the cortex.

Angiosarcoma

These are usually benign capillary or arteriolar malformations. They may involve a vertebra and produce the classical radiological appearance of trabeculae.

An angiosarcoma is a malignant tumour which on X-ray may show areas of calcification. It requires radical excision and sometimes amputation.

Neurofibrosarcoma

These can be single or multiple, as in neurofibromatosis. Neurological deficit may result from pressure on the spinal cord or peripheral nerves. Malignant change is rare and results in a fibrosarcoma. Treatment varies from decompression to radical excision and even amputation.

Malignant Neoplasms

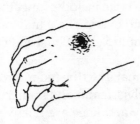

Squamous cell carcinoma

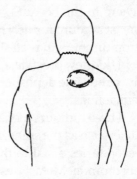

Liposarcoma

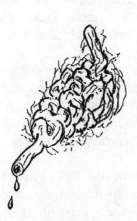

Angiosarcoma

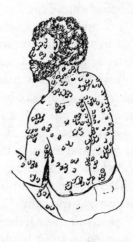

Neurofibrosarcoma

Secondary Neoplasms

Secondary tumours usually arise following blood borne spread from a carcinoma, or occasionally sarcoma elsewhere in the body. Secondaries from carcinoma of the breast account for nearly 50% of metastases. Other common tumours to metastasise to bone include: lung, thyroid, kidney, prostate, cervix and ovary. These may produce multiple deposits, as do multiple myeloma and the leukaemias.

These tumours metastasise mainly to the red marrow areas such as the spine, ribs, pelvis, femur and humerus. Secondaries distal to the elbow and knee are relatively uncommon. Metastases are usually multiple but may be solitary, especially secondaries from the thyroid and kidney, both of which are highly vascular, as are myeloma deposits.

Most secondaries are osteolytic and usually cause punched-out areas, but those from prostate and about 10% of breast secondaries are osteosclerotic. Pathological fractures are common and collapse of vertebrae may occur with paraplegia and quadriplegia.

The diagnosis is made on a history of a primary tumour plus an area of tenderness, pain and perhaps fracture at the site of the metastatic deposit. Many cases, however, first present with a painful area or pathological fracture, and it is only then that a primary tumour is suspected and looked for.

Radiological examination will usually confirm the diagnosis, especially if the existence of a primary tumour is already known. If there is any doubt, a trephine biopsy is carried out but before an anaesthetic or operation is considered a skeletal survey and isotope bone scan should be carried out. The minimum requirements are PA and

Secondary Neoplasms

Common sites for metastases

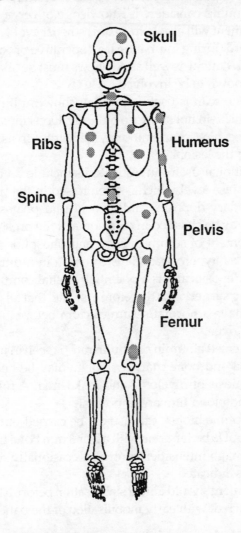

Skull

Ribs

Humerus

Spine

Pelvis

Femur

lateral views of the chest, lateral views of the cervical and lumbar spines, and AP views of pelvis and both humeri and femora. This is important as bones with a potential for pathological fractures may be discovered and prophylactic pinning considered. Knowledge of cervical spine involvement will also help an anaesthetist avoid damage to the cord during intubation if an operative procedure is required. Lateral as well as AP views must be taken of all bones known to be involved.

A bone scan is useful and may show multiple 'hot' areas which do not show up on X-ray. Occasionally a CT or MRI scan or tomogram may be helpful to assess the extent of the lesion.

Additional useful investigations include an alkaline phosphatase level which is often raised in the presence of secondary deposits, and an acid phosphatase level, which may be elevated in carcinoma of the prostate. The measurement of serum calcium and phosphorus is important, as hypercalcaemia is common in multiple secondary deposits and is a potentially lethal complication following surgery. It is therefore essential that all patients should have a normal serum calcium before an anaesthetic is given.

A reversed albumin/globulin ratio is seen in multiple myeloma and bone marrow biopsy may be helpful in the diagnosis of myeloma and leukaemia. A full blood count and blood film are important.

A trephine biopsy can usually be carried out with a needle, but is better done with a 2 or 3 mm bone trephine under image intensifier control. Occasionally an open biopsy is indicated.

Treatment should aim at stabilisation before a fracture has occurred, with early mobilisation of the patient. The

Secondary Neoplasms

Diagnosis

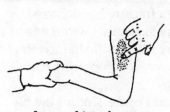

Area of tenderness

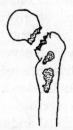

X-ray appearance of a pathological fracture

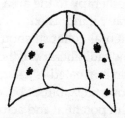

X-ray appearance of secondary deposits

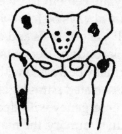

Skeletal survey of painful bones

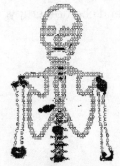

Bone scan

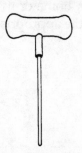

Instrument for trephine biopsy

appropriate general treatment is usually local radiotherapy, plus hormones, such as tamoxifen for breast secondaries and chemotherapy for multiple myeloma, renal and other secondaries.

Stabilisation of the spine, lower humerus, radius, ulna, lower femur and tibia before a fracture has occurred, is usually by the use of a brace or skelecast. Metastases to the pelvis require radiotherapy and those to the acetabulum require skin traction and non-weightbearing mobilisation on crutches.

Potential and actual fractures of the *shaft* of the humerus and femur are best treated with prophylactic and therapeutic internal fixation, together with methyl methacrylate cement to give extra stability if necessary. This must always be followed by radiotherapy to the area as well as hormones and chemotherapy if indicated.

Secondary deposits with vertebral collapse should normally be treated with a brace and radiotherapy. If there is associated paraplegia this should be treated as a surgical emergency with decompression and stabilisation.

In summary, the management of potential and actual pathological fractures aims to stabilise the fracture by the simplest method, enabling the patient to be mobile and return home or to a nursing home as soon as possible after the appropriate radiotherapy and chemotherapy.

Secondary Neoplasms

Treatment

Upper limb and spine

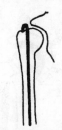

X-ray appearance of a Rush nail

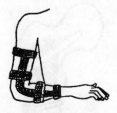

Lower humerus skelecast

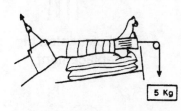

Acetabulum: Russell traction

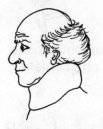

Cervical spine — neck collar

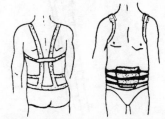

Thoracic spine: Taylor brace

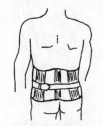

Lumbar spine support

Secondary Neoplasms

Treatment

Lower limb

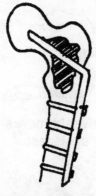

Hip blade plate and cement

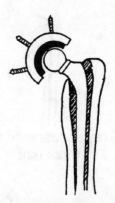

Total cemented hip replacement

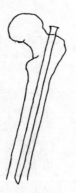

Küntscher nail

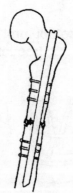

Huckstep titanium locking nail

Chapter 9

Infection

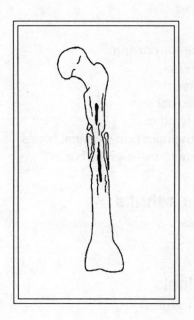

Classification

Osteomyelitis

Acute
Diagnosis
Treatment
Conservative
Medical
Operative

Subacute or chronic
Diagnosis
Treatment
Medical
Operative
Treatment for non-essential bones
Treatment for essential bones

Pyogenic arthritis
Diagnosis
Treatment

Tuberculosis
Clinical features
Investigations
Treatment
Complications

Musculoskeletal Infection

Common sites of occurrence

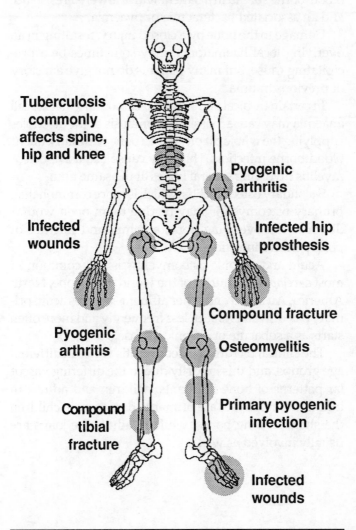

Tuberculosis commonly affects spine, hip and knee

Pyogenic arthritis

Infected wounds

Infected hip prosthesis

Compound fracture

Pyogenic arthritis

Osteomyelitis

Compound tibial fracture

Primary pyogenic infection

Infected wounds

Osteomyelitis

Primary osteomyelitis, or infection of the bone, is usually caused by a pyogenic organism. It is commonly due to blood-borne spread in a patient with a lowered resistance and an associated bacteraemia or pyaemia.

Damage to the bone by a closed injury, resulting in an overlying local haematoma, may sometimes be a precipitating cause, but many patients do not give a history of previous trauma.

In certain tropical and sub-tropical countries sickle cell anaemia may cause massive thrombosis of the arterioles supplying the whole diaphysis of a bone with subsequent blood borne infection. This may cause extensive osteomyelitis involving several bones at the same time.

Secondary osteomyelitis, which is more common than primary osteomyelitis may be due to an open wound down to the overlying bone, a compound fracture or postoperative infection.

Acute and chronic osteomyelitis is still common in most *developing* countries of the world. In Europe, North America, Australia and other affluent societies acute primary osteomyelitis is seen less frequently and more often starts as a subacute or chronic disease.

The clinical picture of osteomyelitis varies in different age groups, and this is partly due to the differing vascular patterns of bone in infants, children and adults. In infants the epiphyses are primarily damaged, in children the shafts of long bones, while in adults the joints are usually involved as well.

Osteomyelitis — Causes

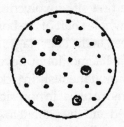

Blood-borne spread

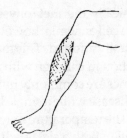

Overlying haematoma

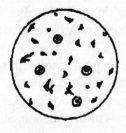

Sickle cell anaemia

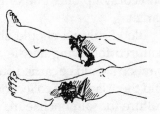

Open wound

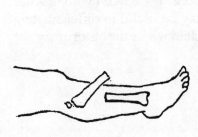

Compound fracture

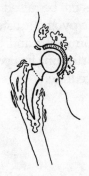

X-ray appearance of an infected prosthesis

Acute osteomyelitis

Diagnosis

Classically the metaphysis is the first site involved. In sickle cell anaemia, however, the whole shaft of the bone is usually affected. This may be seen in the later stages of infection in children with a normal haemoglobin. Several bones are commonly involved simultaneously in sickle cell disease while a single bone is more usual in non-sicklers. The temperature may be raised and the patient toxic and ill in both a sickle cell crisis as well as in acute septicaemic osteomyelitis in the non-sickler.

Classically, evidence of acute osteomyelitis does *not* show radiologically until two to three weeks after the onset of symptoms, but X-ray changes may be seen much earlier.

Blood cultures should always be performed and pus cultured following needle aspiration. Percutaneous aspiration should be carried out if open operation is delayed and there is a large collection of pus under tension. Stool culture for salmonellae may also be useful when sickle cell anaemia is a possibility. The white count may sometimes *not* be raised in salmonella osteomyelitis and low grade pyogenic osteomyelitis. The ESR is raised in acute osteomyelitis and this may be useful in differentiating acute trauma in a young child where the history may not be accurate.

Osteomyelitis

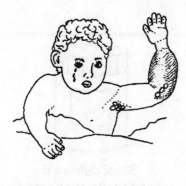

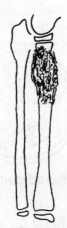

Symptoms and signs: swelling, pain, pyrexia, erythema and lymphadenopathy

X-ray appearance of primary osteomyelitis

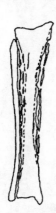

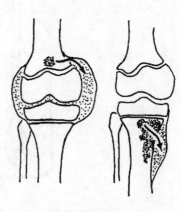

X-ray appearance of osteomyelitis of the tibia

Local spread

Osteomyelitis — Investigations

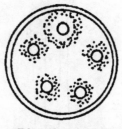

Blood culture

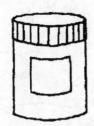

**Stool culture if
salmonella suspected**

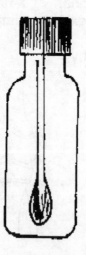

Pus swab in culture media

Osteomyelitis — Investigations

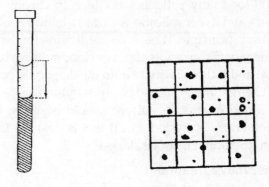

ESR

WBC: total and
differential counts

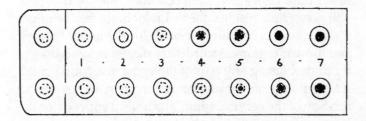

Widal and brucella
agglutination tests

General treatment

It is essential that treatment be *immediate*, *adequate* and *uninterrupted* for at least 1 month and usually longer. There are still too many patients who develop chronic osteomyelitis, and its complications, due to a failure to observe this simple principle. There is no justification for deferring treatment until the results of pus or blood cultures become known and if there is doubt as to the diagnosis, prophylactic chemotherapy should be given *intravenously* in any case. Blood or pus for culture should be taken before chemotherapy is started, but if this is delayed for any reason, treatment must be started.

Conservative treatment

Immobilisation

The splinting of an infected bone is essential as pathological fractures are common and the limb must be rested. A *well padded* plaster back slab (not complete plaster) or a Thomas splint should be used initially and completed as the swelling subsides. An infected upper limb should be elevated in a sling or abduction splint and the lower limb kept elevated in bed. Infections of the spine will necessitate rest in either a Taylor brace for the upper thoracic region or a lumbar brace for the lower thoracic and lumbar regions. An ordinary plaster jacket is useless for immobilising any part of the spine in a young child. A Minerva, or similar support which prevents flexion and rotation of the cervical spine, and a spica support for the lower spine, may be required.

Medical treatment

Antibiotic therapy

High dose, intravenous penicillin or cloxacillin given with probenecid is the best empirical therapy until culture

Osteomyelitis — Treatment

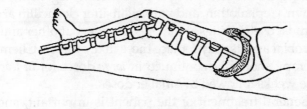

Rest and elevation

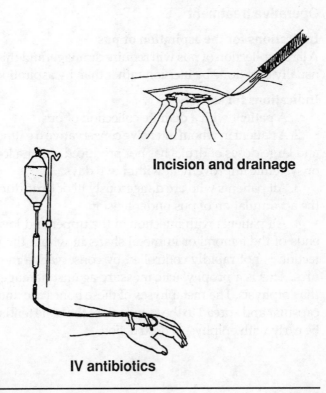

Incision and drainage

IV antibiotics

---

results are known, provided there is no history of penicillin allergy.

This combination of drugs should be changed if necessary once the sensitivity of the infecting organisms is known. Cephalothin, and ampicillin after cloxacillin are the most useful drugs at the present time, but other antimicrobial agents may replace these in the future. Chemotherapy should be continued in *large* doses for *at least* three weeks followed by smaller doses.

General treatment of the patient is important, and blood transfusion may be required for anaemia, particularly in postoperative osteomyelitis.

Operative treatment

Indications for the aspiration of pus
A large collection of pus will require drainage, and this is usually best done by incision rather than by aspiration.

Indications for surgery
1. A patient with a definite collection of pus.

2. A patient in whom intensive conservative treatment and large doses of drugs has not produced either a local or systemic improvement within two days.

3. All patients who are dangerously ill or toxic due to the accumulation of pus under tension.

4. All patients with infection of the upper and lower ends of the femoral or humeral shafts in whom the infection is not rapidly controlled by conservative measures. This is a prophylactic measure against damage to the epiphysis. The metaphyses of these bones are intracapsular and spread to the epiphysis of the bone tends to be early with epiphyseal destruction.

Osteomyelitis — Indications for Surgery

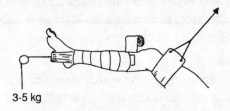

3-5 kg

Failed conservative treatment

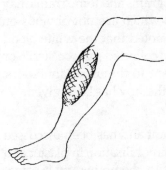

Collection of pus

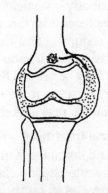

X-ray appearance of infection of intracapsular sites

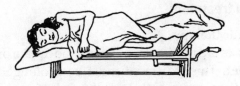

Very ill or toxic patient

Subacute and chronic osteomyelitis

There are many thousands of cases of subacute or chronic osteomyelitis due to incomplete treatment of the acute disease or secondary infection of fractures and bone operations. Osteomyelitis may also start as a subacute or chronic infection without apparent cause.

Diagnosis

The diagnosis is straightforward, except in certain cases of low grade osteomyelitis, chronic infections of the spine and certain atypical cases.

Specific tests which may be helpful are staphylococcal antibody investigations for both the antihaemolysin and antileucocidin titres. Sinograms and tomograms may show sequestra and cavities which are not obvious on ordinary X-ray. It should be noted that the white blood count may be normal, the pus collected may be sterile or the organism may be resistant to the usual antibiotics, especially if previous chemotherapy has been given.

General treatment

Rest and splintage is important and has been discussed under acute osteomyelitis. Immobilisation in plaster and treatment as an outpatient with chemotherapy is sometimes a matter of necessity.

The patient with long standing osteomyelitis may be anaemic and will often benefit from a blood transfusion.

Medical treatment

Antibiotic therapy

Antibiotics are used as an adjunct to adequate operative treatment. This treatment must be prolonged, never shorter than one month and often of several months' duration. In cases where the organism is resistant to all

---

antibiotics or the pus proves to be sterile on culture, cloxacillin may be of value after an adequate sequestrectomy or debridement. Repeated cultures and sensitivities are important and the appropriate antibiotics should be used. The laboratory should be used merely as a guide to the appropriate chemotherapy. Clinical response, side effects, ease of administration and cost are the main guidelines as to the appropriate choice of drugs.

Antibiotic therapy must be prolonged but most antibiotics have side effects if given for long periods. They also have the disadvantage of having to be given 2–4 times per day. In addition, in chronic osteomyelitis avascular bone receives relatively little, or none, of the circulating antibiotic.

Cloxacillin is probably the best antibiotic at the present time, but will probably be superseded in the future.

Operative treatment

This is essential in many cases, but the correct timing and type of operation is important. The surgical management of the various types of subacute and chronic osteomyelitis will be discussed. This treatment is, of course, in *addition* to adequate chemotherapy, splinting and rest.

Chronic osteomyelitis in a non-essential bone

This includes the upper three-quarters of the fibula, the small bones of the hands and feet, the clavicle, some tarsal bones and, in adults, the lower end of the ulna.

In all these bones excision of the focus should be carried out for established infection. Care must be taken, however, in excising part of the fibula in growing children, as a later valgus deformity of the ankle may occur. Implantation of the lower resected end of the fibula into the tibia may prevent this.

Chronic osteomyelitis in essential bones

Sequestra and adequate skin cover.

The following regimen is usually indicated:

1. Sequestrectomy, but *only* when there is adequate involucrum to stabilise the bone.

2. Removal of as much involucrum and avascular bone as possible in order to effect a primary skin closure. Dense scar tissue may also harbour infection.

3. Saucerisation, which involves the surgical excision of tissue, in this case bone, thereby forming a shallow depression with the aim of facilitating drainage of the affected area.

4. Secondary or loose closure of the wound.

5. Adequate splinting and postoperative suction drainage.

Chronic Osteomyelitis

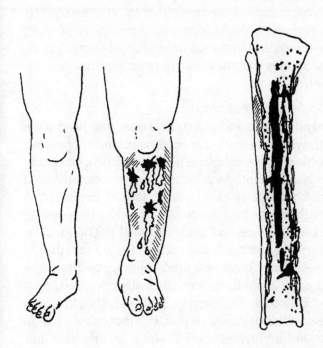

Multiple sinuses

X-ray appearance of sequestra, involucrum and cloacae

Pyogenic Arthritis

Pyogenic arthritis may be primary or due to blood stream spread from another focus. It is sometimes, but not always, associated with an injury of the joint.

It is commonly secondary either to an osteomyelitis involving bone with an intracapsular metaphysis (upper and lower ends of humerus or femur), or from an overlying wound which may or may not communicate with the joint.

Diagnosis and treatment

An early diagnosis and pus culture is essential and acute arthritis will necessitate immediate aspiration of pus and an injection of crystalline penicillin or appropriate antibiotics into the joint space. Washing out the joint through an arthroscope may also have a place in treatment. A pressure bandage over cottonwool may also be required. In the case of knees and ankles, Russell traction will be necessary in order to distract and rest the joint for the hip and knee. Other joints will need splinting and rest. Repeated early aspiration, or occasionally operation, may also be indicated. The incision, however, should *always* be closed after drainage of pus, but there is a place in severe joint involvement for closed joint irrigation and drainage with the appropriate antibiotics, as in osteomyelitis. There is little place for incision and open drainage in most cases as there is with osteomyelitis of the shaft of the bone.

In joint destruction, arthrodesis may be necessary later and occasionally an arthroplasty. In a child this may interfere with growth and should be delayed if possible. Deformities can often be corrected by skin traction alone followed by immobilisation in plaster or a plastic splint.

Pyogenic Arthritis — Causes

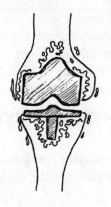

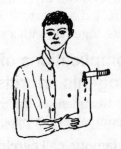

X-ray appearance of an infected knee prosthesis

Penetrating wound

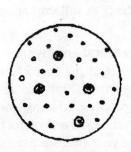

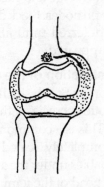

Haematogenous spread

Secondary to osteomyelitis

The joint may subsequently progress to ankylosis without operation and its position should therefore be as functional as possible when this happens.

In the case of severe deformity of the hip, in adults, arthrodesis may be indicated. In children, however, shortening of the limb and recurrence of deformity may occur after operation and this may necessitate a later corrective osteotomy. This is preferable, however, to a gross untreated contracture which may cause a strain on other joints, together with a scoliosis or other deformities.

Complications of osteomyelitis and pyogenic arthritis

The treatment of the more important complications of osteomyelitis and pyogenic arthritis are the following:

Squamous cell carcinoma

This is uncommon and may only occur after several years of discharge from a chronic sinus. Increased pain, a foul discharge and haemorrhage suggest the onset of malignant change and metastases may spread to the draining lymph nodes. Block dissection of glands, however, should be deferred until all the effects of inflammation have disappeared.

Destruction of the upper femoral epiphysis

Thomas Smith, in 1874, discussed the first 21 cases of 'septic necrosis' of the epiphysis of the hip joint in infancy. This is a common complication of late untreated and incompletely treated osteomyelitis and arthritis of the hip in babies under the age of one year. In cases treated early the head of the femur may reform. Diagnosis is by aspiration of pus and definitive operative drainage may be urgently required.

Pyogenic Arthritis

Diagnosis

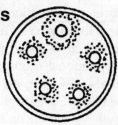

Blood culture

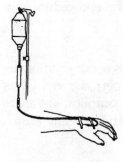

**X-ray appearance of
joint aspiration**

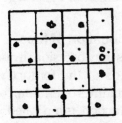

**WCC: total and
differential counts**

Treatment

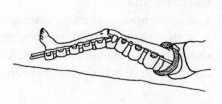

IV antibiotics   **Rest and elevation**

In late cases, with disappearance of the femoral head, an arthroplasty may be necessary in adults. In young children implantation of the upper end of the fibula to replace the upper end of the femur may be performed. In an older child an arthrodesis, shelf operation or sub-trochanteric osteotomy may be the best procedure. Many patients, however, do remarkably well with merely a raised boot. Surgery should, therefore, be deferred until growth has ceased, unless there is extensive deformity or an implantation operation is considered. Total hip replacement may be a good option in the quiescent adult case.

Dislocation of hips

This may occasionally occur instead of destruction of the heads of the femur. Manipulative replacement and sometimes operation, followed by a bilateral hip spica in abduction, is indicated.

Destruction of the lower femoral epiphysis

This may lead to marked valgus or other deformities of growth and requires corrective osteotomy. Recurrence is likely and later stapling to prevent excessive growth on the growing side of the epiphyseal plate can be performed, although osteotomy is probably the best procedure once growth has ceased.

Conclusions

Early diagnosis and immediate intravenous chemotherapy in large doses for prolonged periods, as well as drainage if indicated, are essential if complications are to be minimised, in both osteomyelitis and pyogenic arthritis.

Osteomyelitis and Pyogenic Arthritis

Complications

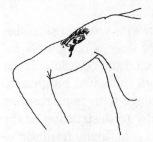

Development of squamous cell carcinoma in chronic sinus tract

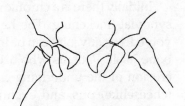

X-ray appearance of destruction of femoral head (Tom Smith's disease)

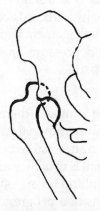

X-ray appearance of a dislocated hip

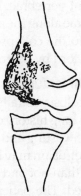

X-ray appearance of epiphyseal destruction; may produce bone growth abnormalities

Tuberculosis

Tuberculosis (TB) of the bones and joints is usually due to infection by the human strain of mycobacterium tuberculosis. It usually spreads from a focus in the lungs, and occasionally from other sites to a joint or the spine, and establishes a chronic infection.

Initially there is a chronic synovitis with considerable synovial thickening. The hip or knee is commonly involved, but any joint can be infected and occasionally the bone itself. Patients who are left untreated progress to erosion of the underlying cartilage with frank caseous (cheeselike) pus, and eventually to destruction of the adjacent bone. Tuberculosis of a joint finally results in fibrous rather than bony ankylosis, unless secondary pyogenic infection is superimposed.

The infection in the spine usually starts at the anterior margins of the vertebrae, adjacent to the disc, with involvement and narrowing of at least one disc and its adjacent vertebrae. Pus can also spread to the adjacent vertebrae along the anterior longitudinal ligament which leads to the collapse of vertebrae and pressure on the spinal cord by necrotic bone or disc tissue.

Clinical features

Tuberculosis usually only affects one joint and there is often a long history of swelling with fairly minimal pain. Muscle wasting and synovial thickening are marked and a joint effusion may be present. The joint is usually warm rather than hot and the regional lymph nodes are often involved. The patient often complains of a progressive deformity, sometimes over a period of months or years, with marked limitation of movement, finally resulting in a fibrous union of the joint.

Tuberculosis

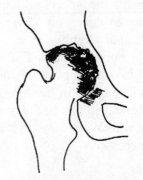

X-ray appearance of hip joint destruction

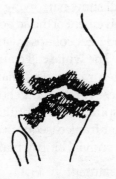

X-ray appearance of knee joint destruction

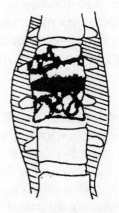

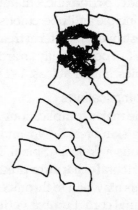

X-ray appearance of destruction of vertebral bodies and intervertebral discs

Investigations

An X-ray may show soft tissue swelling, bone rarefaction and gradual narrowing and destruction of the joint space as the cartilage and bone are involved. The spine will show narrowing of one or more disc spaces with involvement of the adjacent vertebra, an abscess on AP view, and later collapse with production of a kyphos.

The white cell count is usually normal, but the ESR is often raised. The Mantoux test is usually positive and chest X-ray often shows a primary focus in the lungs. Aspiration of joint fluid may show acid fast bacilli and later frank caseous pus. Culture will take 3–6 weeks and a synovial biopsy may also be necessary.

Treatment

Early treatment includes rest of the joint with a splint, or skin traction if the hip and knee are involved. This should progress to non-weight bearing with crutches. Treatment with antituberculous drugs may be prolonged. At present various combinations of rifampicin, isoniazid, pyrazinamide, pyridoxine, ethambutol and streptomycin are the principle antituberculous drugs in use. If a major joint is destroyed, long term treatment options include arthrodesis, or occasionally an arthroplasty if the disease has been quiescent for at least 1–2 years.

Complications

The major complications are secondary infection following skin breakdown, and joint destruction leading to fibrous ankylosis. Spinal TB may cause paralysis due to vertebral collapse or pressure by pus, bone or disc tissue. This may lead to thrombosis of the vessels supplying the spinal cord. Lumbar vertebral infection may track down the psoas sheath producing a psoas abscess in the groin.

Chapter 10

Arthritis

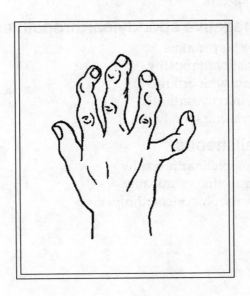

Classification

Osteoarthritis

Rheumatoid arthritis
Still's disease

Crystalline arthropathy
Gout
Pseudogout

Seronegative spondyloarthropathies
Reiter's syndrome
Psoriatic arthropathy
Enteropathic arthritis
Post-infective arthritis
Ankylosing spondylitis

Miscellaneous
Haemophilic arthropathy
Neuropathic arthropathy
Hypertrophic osteoarthropathy

Arthritis

Common sites of occurence

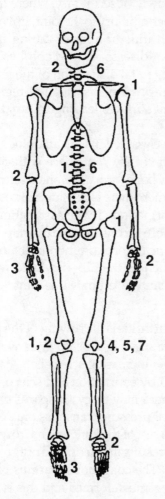

1. Osteoarthritis
2. Rheumatoid arthritis and Still's disease
3. Gout
4. Pseudogout
5. Reiter's syndrome
6. Ankylosing spondylitis
7. Haemophilic arthropathy

Osteoarthritis

Osteoarthritis is a degenerative or 'wear and tear' arthritis which is by far the most common of all the arthritides. It may be primary, usually occurring in the elderly and where the cause is unknown, or secondary, where there is a precipitating cause such as injury to the joint, previous infection, rheumatoid arthritis or a factor dating from childhood such as Perthes' disease, slipped epiphysis or incompletely treated congenital dislocation of the hip.

In secondary osteoarthritis there is usually irregularity of the congruous joint surfaces leading to rapid degenerative changes.

Osteoarthritis may be classified into an atrophic type, where there is diminution of the joint space with cystic spaces and not much new bone formation, and a sclerotic and hypertrophic type where there is considerable osteophyte and new bone formation. This classification is, however, empiric and there is considerable overlap. Primary osteoarthritis is much more common in the main weight-bearing joints such as the hip and knee while secondary osteoarthritis may affect only one joint.

Pathology

The first change in osteoarthritis is narrowing of the joint space, usually at the site of weight-bearing, as well as irregularity and gradually increasing sclerosis.

This is often followed by eburnation and sclerosis of the underlying bone. There may be cystic spaces under this area due to abnormal pressure transmission. As degeneration continues the rest of the joint will narrow and reactive bone formation results in osteophyte outgrowth at the edges of the joint. The congruous margins of the joint often flatten and become deformed and this is par-

Osteoarthritis — Aetiology

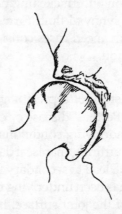

**X-ray appearance of osteoarthritis:
increased incidence with age**

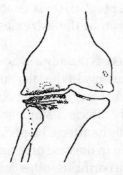

**X-ray appearance of
osteoarthritis secondary
to an old knee fracture**

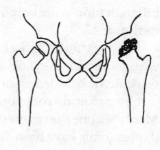

**X-ray appearance of
osteoarthritis
secondary to
childhood Perthes'
disease**

ticularly common in the head of the femur and the lower femoral condyles.

Synovial irritation and thickening occurs in osteoarthritis with excess synovial fluid formed as a result of this synovitis. In advanced cases considerable synovial thickening is common.

Clinical picture

There may be a history of a precipitating condition in childhood such as Perthes' disease or dislocation of the hip. In adult life underlying conditions such as haemophilia, rheumatoid arthritis, meniscal damage or fracture of the patella may all lead to secondary arthritic changes, especially if there has been underlying cartilage damage with incongruity of the joint surface. In many cases no precipitating cause can be found.

Unlike rheumatoid or infective arthritis, primary osteoarthritis is usually slow to progress, with increasing pain, and limitation of joint movement often over a period of years. There is no constitutional upset, pyrexia, or acute inflammation with only mild pain at the extremes of movement.

In osteoarthritis of the knee there is usually a synovial effusion as well as synovial thickening. In the later stage osteophytic broadening of the joint margins may occur.

Osteoarthritis commonly only affects a single joint. More than one joint may eventually be affected especially if other joints have been damaged in the case of secondary osteoarthritis. In primary osteoarthritis, other joints may also have been subjected to abnormal strain, such as back and knee strain accompanying a deformed, stiff, osteoarthritic hip.

Other joints commonly affected in primary osteoarthritis, in addition to the hip and knee, include the spine,

Osteoarthritis — Pathology

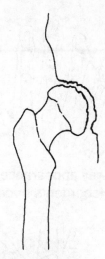

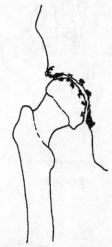

X-ray appearance of degeneration of articular surface

X-ray appearance of loss of joint space and periarticular sclerosis

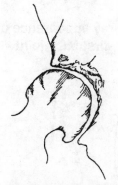

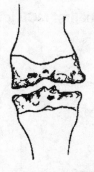

X-ray appearance of severe osteoarthritis: osteophytes, synovial cysts and cartilage denudation

Osteoarthritis — Upper Limb

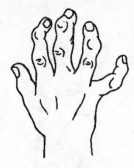

Heberden's
nodes

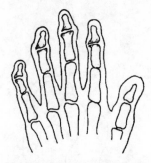

X-ray appearance of
Heberden's nodes

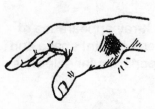

Painful first MCP joint

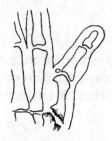

X-ray appearance of
first MCP joint

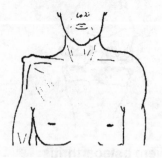

Wasted shoulder

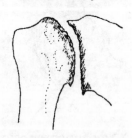

X-ray appearance of
osteoarthritic shoulder

A Simple Guide to Orthopaedics

Osteoarthritis — Lower Limb

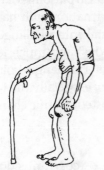

Arthritic gait

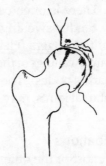

X-ray appearance of an osteoarthritic hip

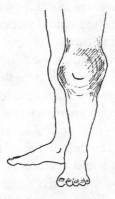

Swollen knee

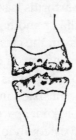

X-ray appearance of knee showing osteophytes

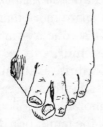

First MTP joint

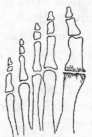

X-ray appearance of first MTP joint

the metatarso-phalangeal joints of the big toes, and the metacarpo-phalangeal and carpometacarpal joints of the thumb. There is often osteophyte formation with hard, slightly tender swellings of the distal interphalangeal joints of the fingers (Heberden's nodes) and much less often hard swellings of the proximal interphalangeal joints (Bouchard's nodes). The small bones, especially the tar-sometatarsal joints, may also show osteoarthritic changes.

Investigations

Unlike most of the other arthritides, osteoarthritis does not cause any constitutional disturbance. In addition, all blood tests and other investigations are normal except where the arthritis is secondary to rheumatoid arthritis, haemophilia or another precipitating cause.

Apart from the classical clinical findings the diagnosis may be confirmed radiologically. Although in the early stages of osteoarthritis X-rays show only slight narrowing of the joint space, in the later stages severe narrowing of the whole joint space may occur, with sclerosis, cystic spaces and osteophyte formation. The destruction of the bone, particularly of the acetabulum and head of the femur, may be severe, with upward subluxation of the head of the femur. In the hip this is usually associated with a deformity in *flexion, adduction* and *external rotation*. Involvement of one side of the joint space more than the other is common in the knee, with a secondary varus or valgus deformity of the tibia or the femur.

X-rays may show that the osteoarthritis is secondary to an underlying condition such as Perthes' disease, a slipped epiphysis, an avascular femoral head following steroid therapy, a fractured neck of the femur or a dislocated hip.

Osteoarthritis — Underlying Conditions

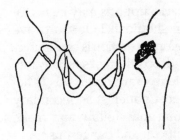

X-ray appearance of
Perthes' disease

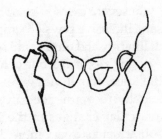

X-ray appearance of
a slipped femoral
capital epiphysis

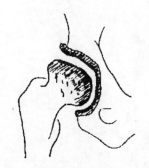

X-ray appearance of
avascular necrosis of the
femoral head

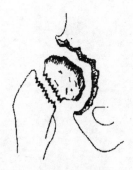

X-ray appearance of
a fracture of the
femoral neck

Conservative treatment

The initial treatment in early osteoarthritis is conservative with analgesics and non-steroidal anti-inflammatory drugs, as well as heat and active exercises. In addition a heel raise will compensate for shortening as well as a flexion deformity of the hip, knee or ankle by preventing excessive stress on the contracted joint when walking.

In severe cases knee or back supports may be necessary. Intensive physiotherapy should include shortwave diathermy and ultrasound before operation is considered. Although local injection of hydrocortisone, especially into the knee, sometimes gives temporary relief, this is not usually recommended in most patients, as secondary avascular changes in the joint may follow and make subsequent surgery more difficult and dangerous.

If there is an underlying cause such as rheumatoid arthritis or gout, this of course should also be treated.

Osteoarthritis — Conservative Treatment

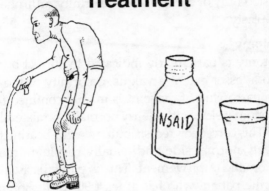

Raised heel and stick

Analgesics and anti-inflammatory medication

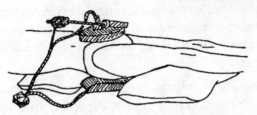

Short wave diathermy

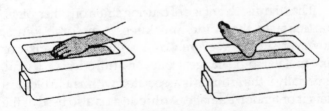

Wax baths and exercises

Operative treatment

The operative treatment of osteoarthritis can be divided into osteotomy or correction of deformity, arthrodesis or arthroplasty.

Osteotomy

Osteotomy is particularly indicated to correct a varus, and to a lesser extent a valgus, deformity of the knee where narrowing of the joint is mainly confined to the inner or outer side, with a fairly normal contralateral joint space. This correction redistributes weight-bearing to the relatively normal side and usually results in marked symptomatic improvement. This is particularly indicated in the patient who has at least 90° of flexion in the affected knee.

Osteotomy in the subtrochanteric region of the hip may also help correct an adduction deformity if there is otherwise a fairly reasonable range of joint movement. It is indicated in patients under the age of forty, but does make subsequent total hip replacement more difficult.

Arthrodesis

Arthrodesis is mainly reserved for a severely osteoarthritic joint with marked destruction, especially in a younger patient when joint replacement is not likely to last, due both to the activity of the patient and the expectation of a relatively long life span.

It has the disadvantage of causing strain on other joints, particularly the spine and knees. In some joints, however, such as a severely osteoarthritic wrist, ankle or first metatarso-phalangeal joint, an arthrodesis is useful, especially if the arthritis is associated with a neurological deficit or tendon damage. Arthrodesis is also used at the knee when a previous total knee replacement has failed.

Osteoarthritis — Operative Treatment

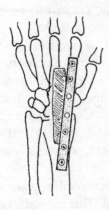

X-ray appearance of a wrist arthrodesis

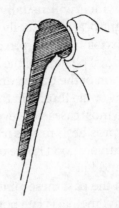

X-ray appearance of a shoulder replacement

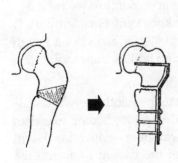

X-ray appearance of a femoral osteotomy

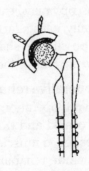

X-ray appearance of a total hip replacement

Arthroplasty

In very unfit patients an excision arthroplasty of the hip, by removing the head and neck of the femur alone (Girdlestone procedure), may result in a painless mobile hip which will usually allow the patient to be fully weight-bearing, usually with the aid of sticks.

Excision of the proximal half to two-thirds of the proximal phalanx of the big toe (Keller's operation) and excision of the trapezium in severe carpometacarpal arthritis of the thumb in the elderly may be indicated.

In most cases, however, replacement of the joint itself by a prosthesis results in a stable and painless joint with a relatively good range of movement, particularly in the hip and knee.

In the past these joints were cemented in place with methyl methacrylate bone cement. This caused loosening, particularly in young patients and as a result, many joint replacements, especially in patients under 55, are now cementless.

Other operations for osteoarthritis

Arthoscopy may be used therapeutically as well as diagnostically, particularly in the knee joint. For example it is often possible to shave the posterior aspect of a rough patella or remove loose foreign bodies from a joint.

Postoperative rehabilitation

Following operation, adequate physiotherapy is usually advocated and this includes strengthening exercises for weakened muscles and walking re-education. It will also include rehabilitation of the patient back into the workforce and home if relevant (Chapter 6).

Osteoarthritis — Operative Treatment

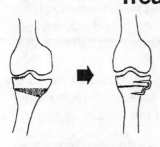

X-ray appearance of a tibial osteotomy

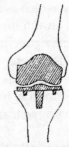

X-ray appearance of a total knee replacement

Postoperative physiotherapy

Shoulder joint

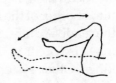

Knee joint

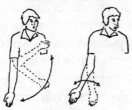

Elbow joint

Hip joint

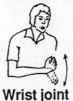

Wrist joint

Ankle joint

Rheumatoid Arthritis

This is a chronic inflammatory polyarthritis of unknown aetiology which is often bilateral and symmetrical. It is probably an autoimmune condition, but other aetiological factors may precipitate it, including an inflammatory process elsewhere.

It is most prevalent in young adults and is three times more common in females than males. Symptoms sometimes first appear in childhood but usually appear at a later age.

Pathologically, there is a chronic proliferative synovitis with villous hypertrophy. The synovium is infiltrated with lymphocytes and plasma cells. A pannus of granulation tissue extends into the joint, gradually eroding the articular cartilage and later, the underlying bone. Cystic spaces may be evident on X-ray. In addition, the overlying tendons and joint capsule may be damaged resulting in tendon rupture or joint ankylosis.

The disease may also be complicated by many extra-articular manifestations, the most characteristic of which are rheumatoid nodules. These commonly occur over the ulnar border of the forearm but they may also occur over the tendo Achillis, sacrum, occiput and sclera. Nodules may also occur in the viscera, particularly the heart and lungs. Other systemic manifestations of the disease include vasculitis, lung disease, Sjögren's syndrome, neurological complications and anaemia.

Clinical course

The disease classically starts in the hands and feet and is usually symmetrical. The metacarpo-phalangeal and proximal interphalangeal joints are initially affected and often the wrists as well. The swellings are warm, fairly

Rheumatoid Arthritis

Common sites of occurrence

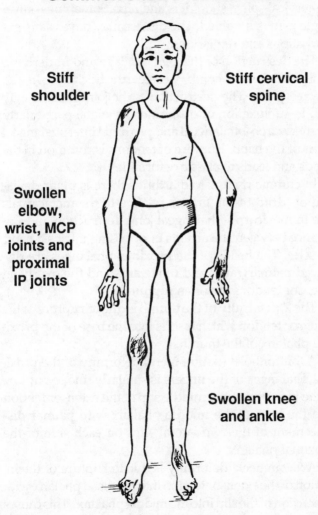

Stiff
shoulder

Stiff cervical
spine

Swollen
elbow,
wrist, MCP
joints and
proximal
IP joints

Swollen knee
and ankle

soft and slightly tender, quite different to the chronic bony hard nodules of the distal interphalangeal joints in osteoarthritis (Heberden's nodes). More proximal joints such as the elbow and knee are often affected as well as the cervical spine, shoulders and hips. Sometimes only a single joint is involved. The disease may have many exacerbations and remissions.

The destruction of the joint cartilage and underlying bone will lead to secondary osteoarthritic changes in the affected joints. The destruction of the joint capsule may lead to subluxation or dislocation of joints, particularly the metacarpo-phalangeal and proximal interphalangeal joints of the hand. Rupture of tendons is common in the hands and leads to classic deformities.

In chronic rheumatoid arthritis there is ulnar deviation or 'drift' of the fingers relative to the metacarpals due to metacarpo-phalangeal joint destruction and imbalance between the actions of opposing intrinsic hand muscles. The heads of the proximal phalanges are displaced palmarwards and ulnawards and the overlying extensor tendons are often ruptured.

The Z deformity of the thumb is due to rupture of the extensor tendon which inserts into the base of the proximal phalanx of the thumb.

A 'buttonhole' (boutonnière) deformity of the proximal phalanges of the fingers is similarly due to rupture of the insertion of the middle slip of the extensor tendon into the base of the middle phalanx with palmar displacement of the two lateral slips on each side of the proximal phalanx.

A 'swan neck' deformity is due to rupture of the insertion of the extensor tendon into the distal phalanx with overaction of the slip into the middle phalanx. This causes

Rheumatoid Arthritis: Upper Limb — Early Changes

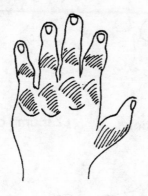

Soft tissue swelling of metacarpophalangeal and proximal interphalangeal joints

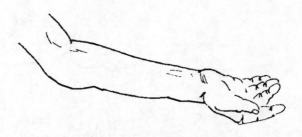

Swollen wrist and elbow

Rheumatoid Arthritis: Upper Limb — Late Changes

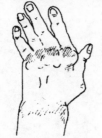

Ulnar deviation

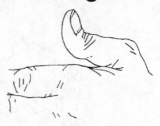

Z thumb deformity

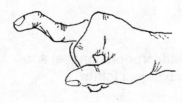

Swan neck deformity

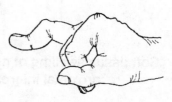

Buttonhole deformity

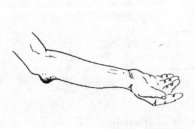

Rheumatoid nodule

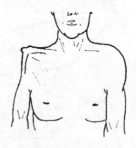

Wasted shoulder

Rheumatoid Arthritis: Lower Limb — Early Changes

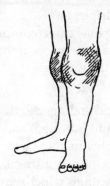

Swollen knees

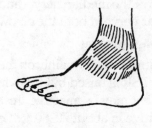

Swollen ankle

Late changes

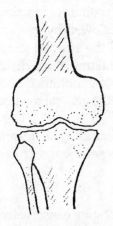

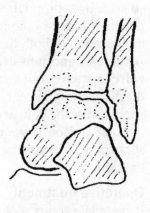

X-ray appearance: destruction of articular surface

a flexed distal phalanx and a hyperextended middle interphalangeal joint.

In severe cases of rheumatoid arthritis marked involvement of the ligaments in the cervical spine may cause subluxation or even dislocation of the vertebrae with neurological changes or even quadriplegia.

In the wrist, synovial thickening may cause compression of the median nerve, and the same may occur to the ulnar nerve at both the elbow and the wrist.

Investigations

Diagnosis relies mainly on the clinical findings discussed. The ESR is raised but the white count is normal and the patient may be anaemic. Tests for rheumatoid factor are positive in about 70–80% of cases but it is not specific to rheumatoid arthritis. Other investigations which may be helpful include complement levels, C-reactive protein, joint aspiration and synovial biopsy.

Conservative treatment

In the acute stages treatment consists of rest of the affected joints by appropriate splints in the 'position of function' plus bed rest for a limited period followed by gradual mobilisation of both the patient and the affected joints. Analgesics and non-steroidal anti-inflammatory drugs will be required, but these should not be continued once the disease is quiescent. Attention to the general medical condition of the patient is important.

Knee and foot supports, walking frames, crutches and sticks may be required to mobilise the patient and protect the skin.

Operative treatment

If synovial proliferation continues, despite conservative management, synovectomy may be required before gross

Rheumatoid Arthritis — Treatment

Conservative

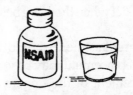

Analgesia and non-steroidal anti-inflammatory drugs (NSAID's)

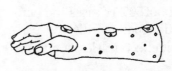

Splint or crepe bandage

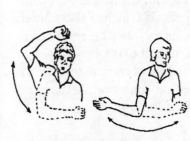

Physiotherapy

Operative

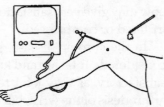

Arthroscopic synovectomy

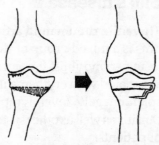

X-ray appearance of an osteotomy

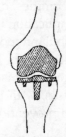

X-ray appearance of a total knee replacement

damage to the articular cartilage has occurred. This may be especially effective in the knees.

Tendon ruptures may require repair or tendon transposition but this should not be carried out in the presence of active disease. Decompression of the median nerve at the wrist, or transposition of the ulnar nerve at the elbow may give very satisfactory relief when these are being irritated or compressed.

In the chronic disease, joint replacement should be considered. Total hip and knee replacement may be very satisfactory, as may joint replacement of the fingers or arthrodesis of the wrist, but only when their *overall* benefit to the patient has been considered.

Still's disease

(Juvenile rheumatoid arthritis)

This is a mixed group of rheumatoid arthritis and ankylosing spondylitis. It occurs in childhood and is usually associated with erythema in about 50% of cases and with splenomegaly, fever, lymphadenopathy, iritis and pericarditis as well as other systemic effects in a lesser number of patients.

There is often stunted growth and in severe cases multiple joint involvement, including the cervical spine with deformities, dislocations and contractures. A common complication is micrognathia which is also known as mandibular hypoplasia or shrew face. This results from involvement of the temperomandibular joints.

The treatment is similar to that of rheumatoid arthritis in adults, with the accent on conservative management and prevention of deformities.

Still's Disease

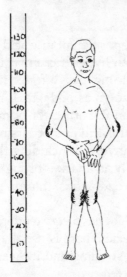

Affected child with stunted growth and involvement of multiple joints

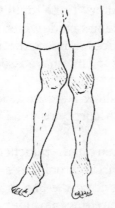

Swollen knees and ankles

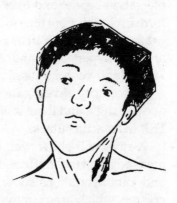

Cervical involvement

Crystalline Arthropathies

Gout

Gout is caused by deposition of uric acid crystals in the joints of patients with hyperuricaemia. The metatarsophalangeal joint of the big toe is affected in about 75% of patients, which is known as podagra. It may be due to either overproduction (inborn error of metabolism), or under excretion of uric acid and occurs mainly in men. Other joints can be involved including the ankle, knee and hands. Classically an attack is brought on by conditions such as stress, operations, trauma or intercurrent infections.

Clinically the patient has a very tender, hot and swollen joint and is pyrexic. There is usually a history of a previous episode of swelling and in over 90% of cases only one joint is affected.

There may be signs of gouty tophi elsewhere especially over the helix of the ear, over the prepatellar and olecranon bursae and over tendons. These tophi which form in chronic gout may ulcerate and exude white chalky urate crystals. These areas may become infected. Patients are often hypertensive and obese and may have associated kidney and vascular disease.

Laboratory investigations show a serum uric acid above 6 mg% and there is often a leucocytosis and raised ESR in an acute attack.

X-rays will show well demarcated, 'punched-out' areas adjacent to the affected joints in chronic cases. Tophi and joint aspirations show classic needle-like uric acid crystals which are negatively birefringent under polarised light.

Gout

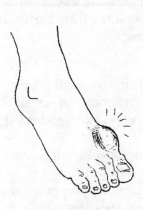

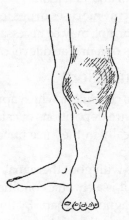

Hot, red, tender swelling of first MTP joint — podagra

Swollen knee

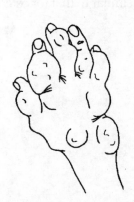

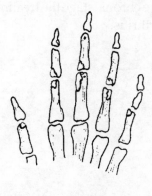

Severe gouty tophi

X-ray appearance of gout

Treatment

In the acute stage a non-steroidal anti-inflammatory drug will usually be sufficient, plus bedrest and avoidance of alcohol and rich food.

In chronic cases drugs to lower the urate level, such as allopurinol, may be necessary, especially if there are renal stones or a uric acid level over 8 mg%.

Pseudogout

In this condition, which appears to have a familial basis, there are depositions of calcium pyrophosphate crystals classically in the knee but also in other joints including the hip.

As with gout there may be acute attacks, but in most cases it is a chronic condition like osteoarthritis.

Diagnosis is made by finding calcium pyrophosphate crystals in the joint aspirate, plus calcification, usually in the menisci of the knee on radiological examination.

Treatment in the acute stage is with joint aspiration, analgesics and non-steroidal anti-inflammatory drugs. In the chronic stage the treatment is similar to that for osteo-arthritis.

Gout

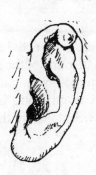

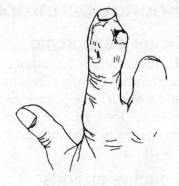

**Gouty tophus in
helix of the ear**

**Gouty tophi with
secondary infection**

Pseudogout

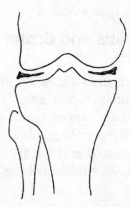

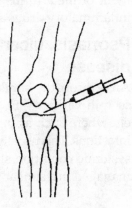

**X-ray appearance of
pseudogout: meniscal
calcification**

**Joint aspiration for
diagnosis**

Seronegative Spondyloarthropathies

Reiter's syndrome

This is classically a triad of arthritis, conjunctivitis and urethritis. It usually affects the small joints of the hands and feet but the hip, knee and other joints may also be affected. The treatment is appropriate antibiotic therapy for the chronic urethritis together with standard therapy for arthritis.

Reactive arthritis

Chronic infections such as chronic osteomyelitis, salmonella, brucella, yersinia enterocolitica and viral infections may cause a non-infective arthritis elsewhere in the body similar to rheumatoid arthritis. This can be treated by addressing the cause, together with conservative management of the arthritis with aspiration and culture, anti-inflammatory drugs and splinting, as required.

Psoriasis, ulcerative colitis and Crohn's disease

An arthropathy similar to rheumatoid arthritis is often seen in various skin, gut and inflammatory conditions elsewhere such as in urogenital and upper respiratory infections. This usually involves the peripheral joints. The systemic condition should be treated and the arthritis managed in a similar fashion to rheumatoid arthritis.

Seronegative Arthritides

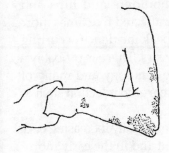

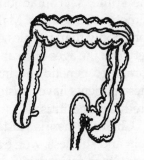

Psoriatic rash on extensor surfaces

Enteropathic arthritis

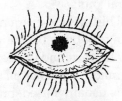

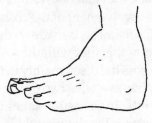

Reiter's disease: conjunctivitis

Reiter's disease: swollen ankle

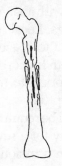

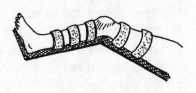

X-ray appearance of chronic osteomyelitis

Splinting for septic arthritis

Ankylosing spondylitis

This is a chronic inflammatory condition affecting mainly the spine, sacroiliac joints, shoulders and hips and sometimes the knees. Males are affected five times more commonly than females, with peak incidence occurring between the ages of 15 and 30 years. There is probably a combined genetic and infective aetiology and many of these patients have a history of chronic infection such as urethritis and iritis.

Clinically there is a history of gradually increasing back pain and stiffness, worse at night and in the early morning. Other major joints may gradually stiffen and the patient has an increasing kyphosis with limitation of all back movements. Limitation of chest expansion is due to involvement of the costo-vertebral joints.

Diagnosis is made on the clinical history and examination together with the X-ray findings of bony bridging across the discs, mainly in the lower thoracic and lumbar spine, as well as narrowing or obliteration of the sacroiliac joints. In the acute stages the ESR is usually raised, but tests for the rheumatoid factor are negative. In over 95% the HLA B27 genetic marker is present.

Treatment is initially conservative, with analgesia and non-steroidal anti-inflammatory drugs. Local heat and back extension exercises are important to prevent a kyphosis. Sleeping on a firm mattress with fracture boards, together with a lightweight back support to maintain extension whilst standing, may be helpful.

Occasionally a hip replacement will be required in the chronic stage as may spinal osteotomy for a severe kyphosis. Low dose radiotherapy has an occasional place for severe unresolved pain.

Ankylosing Spondylitis

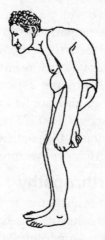

Patient in characteristic posture

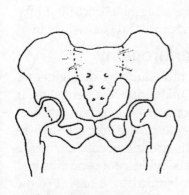

X-ray appearance of reduced sacroiliac joint space

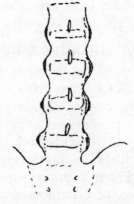

X-ray appearance of a 'Bamboo spine'

Miscellaneous

Haemophilic arthropathy

Haemophiliacs often develop a degenerative arthritis and stiffness in joints, particularly the knee, due to recurrent bleeding and synovitis. In the acute stage it is essential to administer cryoprecipitate before any attempt is made to aspirate the joint. Following aspiration of the joint a pressure dressing should be applied. Care must be taken, as some of these patients are HIV positive as a result of an infected transfusion in the past. In the case of chronic synovitis an arthroscopic synovectomy may be indicated.

Neuropathic arthropathy

Joints with deficient sensation may progress to marked joint destruction and osteoarthritis. In the upper limb this is usually secondary to syringomyelia and the patient may have an abnormally increased range of virtually painless movement of the shoulder despite gross destruction. Similar changes in the lower limb may be due to tertiary syphilis. Occasionally neuropathic joints occur in limbs with denervation such as in spina bifida or in diabetes.

Hypertrophic osteoarthropathy

This is a syndrome of painful clubbing of digits and swelling of the wrists and ankles due to a periostitis. It may occur in pulmonary neoplasms or infection, cyanotic heart conditions or gastrointestinal disorders such as ulcerative colitis, Crohn's disease and hepatic cirrhosis.

Radiologically there may be evidence of periostitis, and dramatic improvement is obtained by removal of the cause i.e. pneumonectomy or even vagotomy.

Miscellaneous Arthritides

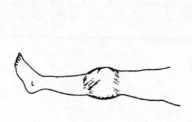

Haemophilic arthropathy

X-ray appearance of secondary osteoarthritis

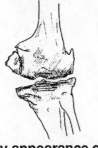

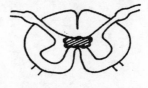

X-ray appearance of a Charcot joint

Neuropathic arthropathy: MRI scan showing syringomyelia

Hypertrophic osteoarthropathy

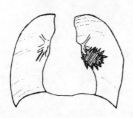

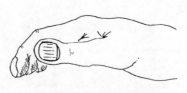

May be secondary to a pulmonary neoplasm

Clubbing of fingers with wrist swelling

Chapter 11

Neurological and Spinal Conditions

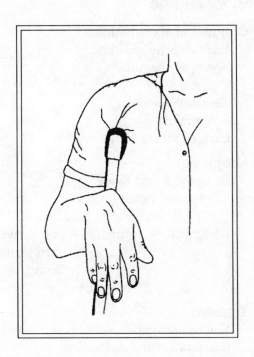

Classification

Cerebral Conditions

Cerebral palsy
Head injuries
Haemorrhage
Thrombosis and embolus
Neoplasms

Spinal Conditions

Cervical spine

Congenital abnormalities

Klippel–Feil syndrome
Sprengel's shoulder
Cervical rib
Torticollis
Spina bifida
Congenital webbing

Neoplasia

Benign —   soft tissue
cartilaginous
bony
Malignant —   primary —   soft tissue
cartilaginous
bony
secondary

Trauma

Soft tissue injuries — tendons / ligaments
Subluxation and dislocation
Fractures

Infection
Discitis
Osteomyelitis
Tuberculosis

Arthritis
Autoimmune — rheumatoid arthritis
                     ankylosing spondylitis
Degenerative — cervical spondylosis

Paralysis
Poliomyelitis
Syringomyelia

Thoracic and lumbar spine

Congenital abnormalities
Spina bifida and meningomyelocele
Lumbarisation and sacralisation of vertebrae
Spondylolysis and spondylolisthesis
Spinal stenosis
Diastematomyelia
Hemivertebrae

Neoplasia
Benign — meningioma
            neurofibroma
            haemangioma
            eosinophilic granuloma
Malignant — primary
               secondary

Trauma
Soft tissue injuries — tendons / ligaments
Subluxation
Dislocation
Fractures

Infection
Discitis
Osteomyelitis
Tuberculosis

Arthritis
Rheumatoid arthritis
Ankylosing spondylitis

Spinal paralysis
Trauma
Thrombosis and embolus of the spinal cord
Neurofibromatosis
Transverse myelitis
Syringomyelia

Scoliosis
Congenital abnormalities
Paralysis
Idiopathic causes
Compensatory

Kyphosis and lordosis
Congenital abnormalities
Neoplasia
Trauma
Infection
Osteoporosis
Paget's disease
Scheuermann's disease

Back pain
Congenital abnormalities
Neoplasia
Trauma

Infection
Prolapsed intervertebral disc
Miscellaneous conditions

Pelvic and Sacral Conditions

Congenital abnormalities

Neoplasia
Benign — soft tissue
cartilaginous
bony
Malignant — primary — soft tissue
cartilaginous
bony
secondary

Trauma
Soft tissue injuries
Subluxation and dislocation
Fractures

Infection
Soft tissue
Bone (osteomyelitis)
Joint (pyogenic arthritis)

Arthritis
Degenerative (osteoarthritis)
Autoimmune (ankylosing spondylitis)

Miscellaneous conditions
Paralysis
Coccydynia

Peripheral Nerve Lesions

Aetiological classification

Peripheral neuritis
Peroneal muscular atrophy
Duchenne muscular dystrophy
Friedreich's ataxia
Poliomyelitis

Anatomical classification

Upper limb nerve lesions

Brachial plexus
Axillary nerve
Radial nerve
Ulnar nerve
Median nerve
Digital nerves
Sudek's atrophy
Nerve entrapment

Lower limb nerve lesions

Cauda equina
Lumbosacral plexus
Sciatic nerve
Common peroneal nerve
Tibial nerve

Peripheral Nerve Lesions
Common sites of occurrence

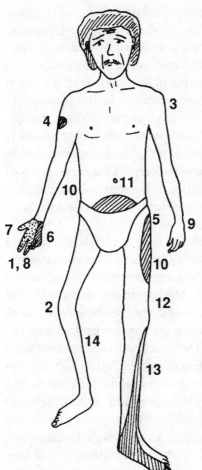

1. Peripheral neuritis
2. Poliomyelitis
3. Brachial plexus
4. Axillary nerve
5. Radial nerve
6. Ulnar nerve
7. Median nerve
8. Digital nerve
9. Sudek's atrophy
10. Nerve entrapment
11. Cauda equina
12. Sciatic nerve
13. Common peroneal nerve
14. Tibial nerve

Introduction

Paralysis may be due to cerebral, spinal or peripheral causes, or to a combination of these. If it is cerebral or spinal *above* the lumbar region, paralysis is usually spastic in nature. Lesions at the lumbar region affecting the cauda equina and peripheral nerves usually cause a flaccid paralysis. In the thoraco-lumbar region there may be a mixture of flaccid and spastic paralysis due to damage to both the lower cord and the cauda equina.

Neurological dysfunction may affect power, sensation and autonomic functions, particularly the bladder. In poliomyelitis, in which the anterior horn cells in the spinal cord are selectively destroyed, only motor power is affected. In peripheral neuritis due to diabetes or certain toxins only sensation may be altered. Common causes of paralysis vary from conditions present at birth, such as spina bifida, to paralysis from tumours, trauma, infections and degenerative conditions.

A detailed examination of the patient should include a thorough evaluation of the peripheral nervous system, including: tone, power, reflexes, sensation, co-ordination and autonomic function. Higher centres and the cranial nerves should also be assessed and the spine itself examined for tenderness, muscle spasm, deformities and cutaneous abnormalities. The examination of a patient with lower back pain or sciatica should include a rectal examination to exclude an intrapelvic lesion where carcinoma of the bladder, prostate, uterus or rectum, or an intrapelvic abscess could be responsible. Abdominal examination should exclude cholecystitis, as well as gastrointestinal, genitourinary, gynaecological, retroperitoneal and vascular causes such as an aortic aneurysm.

Neurological Conditions

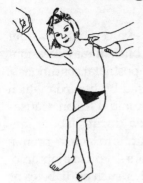

Cerebral palsy

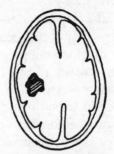

**CT appearance of a
cerebral neoplasm**

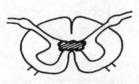

**CT appearance of
syringomyelia**

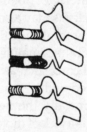

**X-ray appearance
of a prolapsed disc**

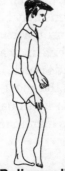

Poliomyelitis

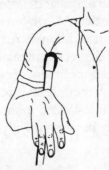

Radial nerve palsy

Cerebral Conditions

Cerebral palsy

Cerebral palsy is a non-progressive cerebral disorder which usually occurs before or at birth. It may occasionally be due to meningitis or other postnatal conditions.

The majority of cases are caused by hypoxia which commonly produces an extrapyramidal lesion. Causes of cerebral palsy include hypoxia during labour, antepartum haemorrhage, pre-eclamptic toxaemia, prematurity or postmaturity of the infant, and cardiopulmonary or other diseases of the mother such as diabetes or renal impairment.

Maternal rubella and rhesus incompatibility with kernicterus may also affect the brain as may birth trauma and cerebral infections such as meningitis. Developmental abnormalities of the brain and occasionally of the spinal cord such as meningomyelocele may also be associated with cerebral damage.

Clinically the neurological dysfunction in cerebral palsy is a lack of motor control. This may be due to defects in the basal ganglia with extrapyramidal signs such as increased tone in muscles. There may be cerebellar signs with ataxia and incoordination, or pyramidal signs with spasticity. A combination of these signs may be present.

In addition there may be some sensory loss and varying degrees of mental retardation. There may also be fits and impairment of sight, hearing and speech.

Although spastic hemiplegia is the most common manifestation, monoplegia, diplegia and quadriplegia may be present with any of the signs mentioned above.

Cerebral Palsy

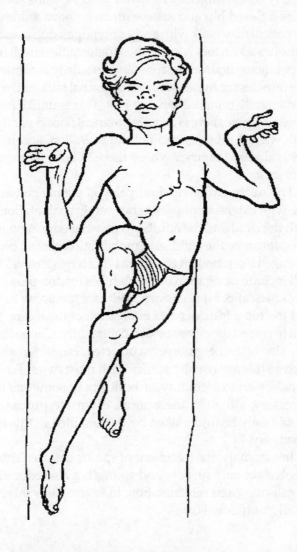

Clinically the patient may present with a flexed elbow and palmar-flexed, pronated wrist with a swan-neck deformity of the fingers. The lower limb or limbs usually show a flexed hip and knee with an equinus ankle and the patient may walk with a scissor type gait due to spasm of the hip adductors. Most of these deformities result from upper motor neurone lesions, and spasticity is common. The muscles are hypertonic and of normal bulk, and there is often only minimal sensory loss. This is unlike poliomyelitis where there is an asymmetrical flaccid paralysis with wasted muscles and normal sensation, and in peripheral nerve injuries where there is both motor and sensory loss.

The treatment of cerebral palsy is mainly conservative with extensive physiotherapy and rehabilitation for both the child and the adult. Intensive re-education may often improve the child, and mobilisation should be encouraged if cerebral involvement is not too extensive. This will include elongation of the Achilles tendon plus a below knee caliper if necessary, adductor tenotomy to correct the hip adductors and elongation of the biceps tendon to correct the elbow flexion contracture. Contractures can also often be passively corrected. Simple methods such as this are usually sufficient in most cases. Tendon transfers and osteotomy of bones may sometimes be necessary, although these more extensive procedures should only be undertaken by those skilled in this type of surgery.

In summary, the treatment of spastic children should involve not only surgery and splints but also education, mobilisation and rehabilitation. In severe cases this may entail institutional care.

Cerebral Palsy — Treatment

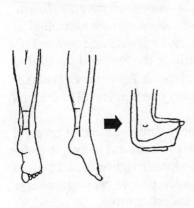

Correction of equinus deformity: elongation of Achilles tendon

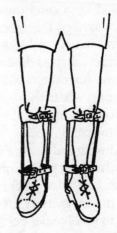

Below knee calipers

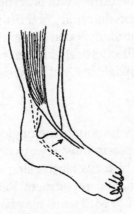

Tendon transfer

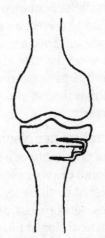

X-ray appearance of an osteotomy

Stroke and head injuries

A stroke is defined as an upper-motor neurone lesion which is often acquired in later life. Stroke is usually caused by a cerebrovascular incident which includes haemorrhage, thrombosis or embolus. It may also follow a head injury, and less commonly various neurological disorders such as disseminated sclerosis and cerebral tumours. A stroke usually affects the arm and leg on the side opposite to the cerebral lesion. As with cerebral palsy, however, it may affect only one limb, or all four limbs and the trunk.

The clinical picture is very similar to that of cerebral palsy with all gradations of physical and mental impairment. Left-sided cerebral lesions in right-handed people and in a majority of left-handed people, cause dysphasia due to involvement of the speech centres.

The treatment is very similar to cerebral palsy with the emphasis being on mobilisation and rehabilitation. Simple subcutaneous elongation of the tendo Achillis alone to correct an equinus deformity will often also reflexly improve a spastic flexion deformity of the hip and knee on the side affected. Similarly, open elongation of the biceps tendon alone will often reflexly improve a palmar flexion and pronation deformity of the wrist and forearm.

Cerebral neoplasms

The possibility of a secondary tumour, a meningioma, a glioma or other cerebral neoplasm must always be considered in all patients with a history of increasing weakness, sensory loss, ataxia or mental impairment. Referral to a neurologist plus EEG, CT or MRI scans may be indicated as well as other investigations.

Stroke and Head Injuries

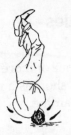

Fall onto head

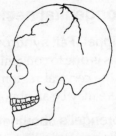

X-ray appearance of a skull fracture

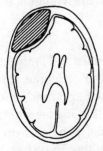

CT appearance of an extradural haemorrhage

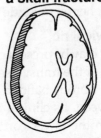

CT appearance of a subdural haemorrhage

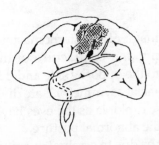

CT appearance of an embolus or thrombus

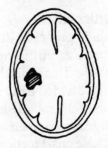

CT appearance of a cerebral neoplasm: primary lesion or secondary deposit

Cervical Spine Conditions

Congenital neck deformities

Klippel–Feil syndrome

This is due to congenital fusion of one or more vertebrae in the cervical region. The neck is short as a result and there may be an abnormally low hairline.

Sprengel's shoulder

This is due to a high-riding scapula on one or both sides. The scapula can be felt to be high and the whole shoulder is higher on one side than the other.

Cervical rib

This may be present on one or both sides and is an extension of the transverse processes of the vertebrae. It may be a fibrous band, a complete rib, or any gradation in between. Its clinical importance is that it may impinge upon the lower cords of the brachial plexus or on the subclavian artery. Very occasionally the rib or band requires excision due to vascular or neurological compression which is usually made worse by downward traction on the arm.

Torticollis

This is probably due to damage of the sternomastoid muscle at birth with swelling and contracture of the muscle. This pulls the head to the opposite side and if it is not divided early leads to facial asymmetry. Late division of the muscle may cause diplopia as the eyes have gradually compensated for the abnormal posture.

Late onset torticollis may be due to cerebral or spinal conditions including injuries of the cervical spine. Spasmodic torticollis sometimes has a psychological cause.

Cervical Spine — Congenital Abnormalities

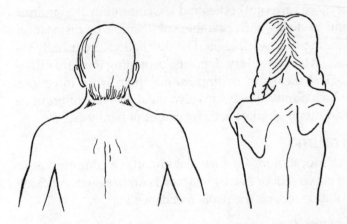

Klippel–Feil syndrome

Sprengel's shoulder

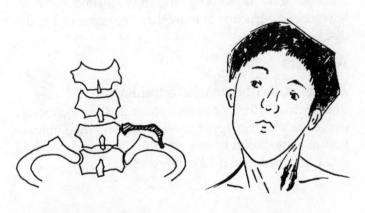

**X-ray appearance
of a cervical rib**

Torticollis

Neoplasia

Secondary deposits in the vertebrae are the most common cause of neurological compression. These affect one or more vertebral bodies and less commonly the laminae and pedicles with possible subluxation or dislocation leading to quadriplegia. The disc spaces are usually intact, with secondary deposits, providing a useful radiological means of distinguishing them from infections which almost always involve the disc. Neurofibromata and meningiomata are rare causes of paralysis.

Trauma

A dislocation or fracture dislocation is a common cause of nerve root or even spinal cord compression. A flexion rotation force is the usual mechanism.

Infection

Pyogenic infection usually involves one disc space alone initially with the adjacent vertebrae. There may also be an abscess which can cause cord compression.

Tuberculous infection is much more insidious and often causes destruction of more than one vertebra and the disc between.

Arthritis

Autoimmune (rheumatoid arthritis)

Rheumatoid arthritis causes softening of the ligaments, particularly in the upper cervical region with subluxation or dislocation of the odontoid peg and possible quadriplegia due to cord compression.

Cervical Spine Conditions

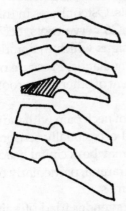

X-ray appearance of a secondary neoplasm

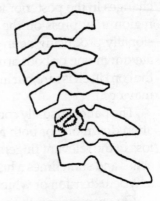

X-ray appearance of a vertebral fracture and dislocation

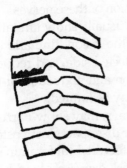

X-ray appearance of discitis

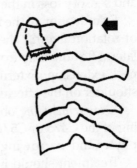

X-ray appearance of the atlas subluxed on the axis

Degenerative (cervical spondylosis)

This condition commonly affects the C4/5 and C5/6 disc spaces with narrowing and secondary degenerative changes in the posterior facet joints. Osteophytes in this region may press on the C5 and C6 nerve roots, occasionally producing neurological signs which may radiate down one or both arms into the hands. Pressure on the cord itself is rare, but involvement of other nerve roots may occur.

The patient usually complains of neck pain with radiation down one or both arms and occasionally sensory loss in the relevant fingers. There may be occipital headaches and sometimes a history of trauma, particularly of a hyperextension or whiplash injuries.

On examination there is often a tender triad of pain over the base of the neck, the insertion of the deltoid and over the extensor muscles of the forearm (not the extensor origin which is referred to as tennis elbow). The biceps jerk may be diminished in a C5 or 6 lesion and the triceps in a C7 or C8 lesion and there may be associated motor and sensory loss in the distribution of these nerves.

Examination of the neck will usually show limitation of rotation *towards* the side of the lesion, limitation of lateral flexion *away* from the affected side, and reduced neck extension. External rotation and abduction of the shoulder on the affected side may be limited.

X-rays, *including* oblique X-rays, may show narrowing of the C4/5 or C5/6 or other disc spaces with osteophytes and narrowing of the intervertebral foramina.

Treatment should include neck exercises, local heat, traction with *rotation* and *flexion* to the side of the lesion, anti-inflammatory drugs, analgesia, and a supportive collar.

Cervical Spine Conditions — Cervical Spondylosis

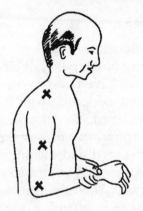

'Huckstep tender triad'

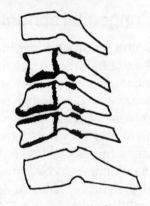

X-ray appearance of
cervical spondylosis

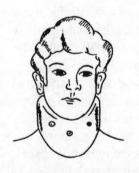

Supportive collar

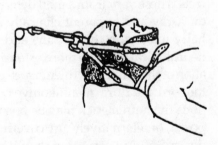

Neck traction with
rotation and flexion to
side of lesion

Thoracic and Lumbar Spine Conditions

Congenital abnormalities

Spina bifida and meningomyelocele

Spina bifida is a congenital defect of the posterior elements in the vertebral arch which have failed to fuse, usually of the lumbar region and associated with involvement of the spinal nerves and cord. Nerve involvement may vary from tethering to protrusion of the meninges (myelocele) or of both the cord and meninges (meningomyelocele). In addition there may be an associated hydrocephalus in severe cases. There is a genetic predisposition, with a 5–10% risk of an offspring being born with spina bifida if a parent or sibling has a similar defect.

Diagnosis in utero may be made by analysis of amniotic fluid for alpha-fetoprotein and ultrasound imaging of the foetus.

Clinical examination may reveal all gradations of defects. These vary from a mild defect which is only evident on X-ray and apparent clinically as a small dimple, or hairy naevus in the midline and not accompanied by neurological signs, to more extensive defects with herniation of the dural sack (meningocele) or herniation of both the cord and dura (meningomyelocele). In severe herniations the hernial sack may be open and the contents exposed, or alternatively any coverings may rapidly break down. Surgical correction should be undertaken as soon as possible.

All gradations of motor, sensory and autonomic impairment may occur, from talipes equino varus to com-

Spina Bifida and Meningomyelocele

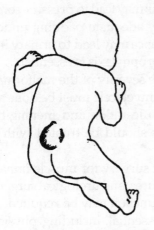

Meningomyelocele

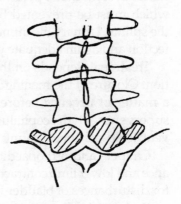

X-ray appearance of spina bifida

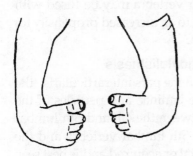

Talipes equino varus

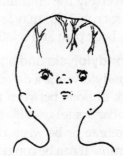

Hydrocephalus

plete paralysis and dislocation of the hips. Bladder paralysis may lead to infection and ascending pyelonephritis.

Motor paralysis varies and is sometimes progressive. It should be treated initially as simply as possible with soft tissue surgery and splinting. Sensory loss in the distribution of the motor paralysis may lead to pressure sores which must be prevented by adequate padding under the splints. Urinary incontinence may lead to urinary infection and again adequate prophylaxis is essential.

Treatment depends on the severity of the malformation. Closure of the meningomyelocele must be done as a matter of urgency before ulceration and meningitis supervenes. Hydrocephalus should be treated with a ventriculo-peritoneal shunt.

Calipers and orthopaedic surgery for muscle imbalance and lower limb contractures, and urological surgery for disturbances of bladder function may be required.

Prolonged follow up is essential, including physiotherapy and rehabilitation.

Lumbarisation and sacralisation of vertebrae

The upper sacrum may form a 6th lumbar vertebra and conversely the 5th lumbar vertebra may be fused with the sacrum. This may lead to an increased propensity for low back pain and sciatica.

Spondylolysis and spondylolisthesis

Spondylolysis is a defect in the pars interarticularis, (the neck of bone between the laminae and pedicles of the lumbar spine) usually between the 4th and 5th lumbar vertebrae or between the 5th lumbar vertebra and the sacrum. It can be congenital or acquired and is best seen on oblique X-rays.

Spondylolisthesis is a forward slip of one vertebra on another, most commonly in the lower lumbar region,

Spondylolysis and Spondylolisthesis

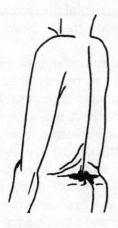

Spondylolisthesis — step in lumbosacral region

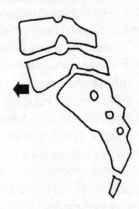

X-ray appearance of a forward slip

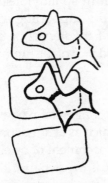

Oblique X-ray: spondylolysis

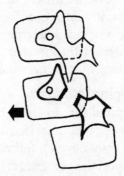

Oblique X-ray: spondylolisthesis with forward displacement

which may result in cauda equina compression. Back pain is common, but neurological signs are uncommon.

The most common cause of a mild spondylolisthesis occurring in any part of the lumbar spine is degeneration of the facet joints and the intervertebral disc secondary to osteoarthritis. Again neurological signs are uncommon, but back pain may be severe.

Clinically, apart from muscle spasm and tenderness of the lower lumbar spine, a step may be felt at the site of a slip as one vertebra and its spinous process subluxes forward on the vertebra below. A defect in the pars inter-articularis seen on *oblique* X-rays has been compared to the head, eyes and ears of a Scottish terrier dog. A collar at its neck signifies a spondylolysis. A forward slip of its head (represented by the transverse process and upper pedicle) on the body and front legs (represented by the lower pedicle and spinous processes) signifies a spondy-lolisthesis. Investigations should include not only X-ray views of the area, but also CT scans of the individual vertebrae and occasionally an MRI scan in addition.

The treatment of back pain in spondylolisthesis is usually back exercises, rest and a supporting corset. In severe cases, decompression of the nerves or postero-lateral arthrodesis of the affected part of the lumbar spine alone may be necessary.

Spinal stenosis

Spinal stenosis may be due to congenital narrowing of the spinal canal in conditions such as achondroplasia or it may develop following encroachment of osteophytes upon the vertebral canal as occurs in osteoarthritis of the facet joints. Alternatively spinal stenosis may be second-ary to a previous fracture of the vertebral bodies. As a result the vertebral canal is narrowed and the patient may develop symptoms of claudication with pain in the calves and yet have a *normal* peripheral circulation.

Diagnosis is by X-ray and CT scan, the latter being safer and more effective than myelography in most cases. Treatment is laminectomy and decompression of the spinal cord.

Diastematomyelia

This is a congenital defect in which the lower spinal cord is divided by a fibrous band or bony spicule. It is often associated with spina bifida and may produce a neurological deficit. It is often progressive during growth of the child.

Hemivertebrae

A congenital defect of part of a vertebra may cause a scoliosis. The spine will obviously be weak and although paraplegia is uncommon a protective corset or an arthrodesis of the spine may be required.

Neoplasia

Meningioma

A meningioma arising from the meninges is a slow growing benign tumour which may cause paraplegia, particularly in the thoracic spine.

Neurofibroma

Neurofibromata are discussed in Chapter 8. A neurofibroma arising from a spinal root in the spinal canal can cause partial or complete paralysis due to pressure on the cord.

Haemangioma

Haemangioma of the vertebra is usually a congential lesion diagnosed on X-ray by coarse striae. It seldom requires treatment except low dose radiotherapy if symptomatic.

Eosinophilic granuloma

Eosinophilic granuloma usually causes complete collapse of the vertebral body and is known as Calve's disease. It is not uncommon in children and young adults and usually does not require operative treatment. Occasionally a more extensive eosinophilic granuloma of the spine will require treatment with low dose radiotherapy.

Trauma

Soft tissue injuries

Soft tissue injuries of the spine are common and are due usually to sudden twisting and flexion strains or to direct trauma. Closed injuries seldom require more than heat, exercise and sometimes a back support.

Subluxation and dislocation

Subluxations and dislocations without a fracture may occur in the cervical spine causing nerve compression and occasionally quadriplegia. The diagnosis and management of these conditions are discussed in 'A Simple Guide to Trauma'.

Fractures

Fractures of the spine can be divided into two categories: stable without displacement with intact posterior ligaments, or those that are unstable. Stable fractures usually present *without* neurological signs and only require rest, back exercises and support.

Unstable fractures usually show displacement of one vertebra on another, often associated with rupture of the interspinous and supraspinous ligaments and most have some neurological deficit. In the thoraco-lumbar and

Thoracic and Lumbar Spine Conditions

Neoplasia

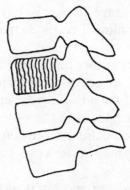

X-ray appearance of a haemangioma

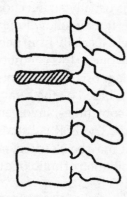

X-ray appearance of an eosinophilic granuloma

Trauma

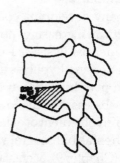

X-ray appearance of a stable fracture of vertebral body

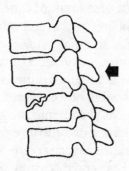

X-ray appearance of an unstable vertebral fracture

cervical regions incomplete unstable lesions may require operative stabilisation.

Infection

Discitis

This is usually an infection of a disc space in the lumbar spine. It may follow lumbar puncture or may be blood borne, especially from pelvic infections. Drug addicts are also prone to this condition.

Diagnosis, apart from clinical history and examination, is based on the X-ray appearance of disc narrowing and, sometimes, involvement of the adjacent vertebral bodies. The ESR is usually raised, the white blood cell count may be elevated, and blood culture taken before the initiation of antibiotic therapy may isolate a pyogenic organism.

Treatment should include bed rest and intravenous antibiotics followed by mobilisation and oral antibiotics for at least three months. Any causative factors should also be treated.

Tuberculosis of thoracic and lumbar spine

Tuberculosis is still common in many developing countries and may cause paraplegia with an increasing motor and sensory deficit as well as bladder paralysis. The onset is usually insidious with an increasing kyphosis and possible abscess formation which may track down the psoas sheath into the groin, if the abscess is in the lower thoracic or lumbar region. There is involvement of at least one disc space and its adjacent vertebrae but several vertebrae and discs may be involved (Chapter 9). Metastatic deposits, on the other hand, usually spare the intervertebral discs.

Thoracic and Lumbar Spine Conditions

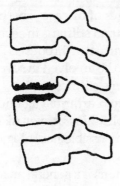

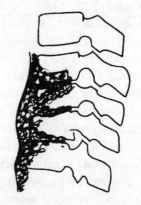

X-ray appearance of discitis

X-ray appearance of spinal tuberculosis

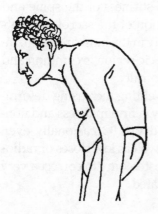

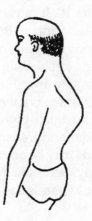

Kyphosis

Kyphos

Arthritis

Rheumatoid arthritis

Rheumatoid arthritis is discussed in more detail in the relevant chapter on arthritis (Chapter 10). It mainly affects the cervical spine in the later stages of disease. There is usually considerable osteoporosis and stiffness in severe cases and this may progress to a virtual arthrodesis. The thoracic and lumbar spine can also be involved in severe cases and be osteoporotic with some stiffness.

In the early stages of rheumatoid arthritis, ligamentous laxity may allow forward subluxation or even dislocation of the atlas on the axis with possible neurological pressure and even quadriplegia.

This can be particularly hazardous if a general anaesthetic is necessary, as intubation may cause subluxation or dislocation with paralysis.

Ankylosing spondylitis

Ankylosing spondylitis is discussed in more detail in Chapter 10. It causes marked stiffness of the spine and sacroiliac joints with obliteration of the sacroiliac joints and bony bridging, particularly in the lumbar region. Increasing kyphosis in the thoracic region is common and may lead to a very severe deformity.

Treatment is aimed at preventing increasing deformity by adequate physiotherapy, a firm mattress and non-steroidal anti-inflammatory drugs. Occasionally even steroids may be necessary as well as low doses of radiotherapy. Occasionally spinal osteotomy to correct a very severe kyphosis may be indicated.

Thoracic and Lumbar Spine Conditions — Paralysis

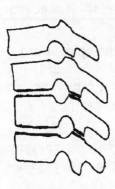

X-ray appearance of spinal rheumatoid arthritis

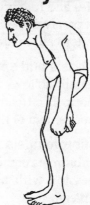

Ankylosing spondylitis

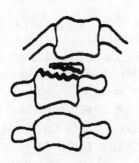

Paralysis may be secondary to spinal trauma

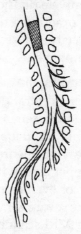

Thrombosis of vessels supplying the spinal cord

Spinal Paralysis

Trauma

Fractures and fracture dislocations may cause all gradations of paralysis (see above). In addition penetrating injuries often cause paralysis.

Thrombosis and embolus of the spinal cord

This usually follows trauma and occasionally infection
or tumour. The treatment is of the cause together with
the management of the associated paraplegia.

Neurofibromatosis

Neurofibromata of the spinal nerve roots may cause cord
compression with partial or complete paraplegia or
quadriplegia.

Transverse myelitis

This is probably due to a viral infection and usually results
in complete division of the spinal cord with paraplegia
and sometimes quadriplegia. Treatment of musculoskeletal paralysis, sensory loss and bladder involvement
is symptomatic.

Syringomyelia

This is a central degeneration of the spinal cord, most
commonly seen in the cervical region. The sensory components are usually involved more than the motor.
Charcot type neuropathic joints may occur, especially in
the upper limb, with little or no pain and often an appreciable or even increased range of movement which be-
lies the severe X-ray changes. Diagnosis is confirmed on
CT or MRI scanning of the affected spinal cord. Treatment is symptomatic.

Thoracic and Lumbar Spine Conditions — Paralysis

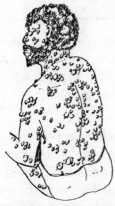

Neurofibromatosis may be complicated by spinal paralysis

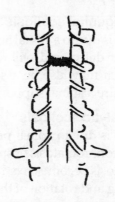

Transverse myelitis

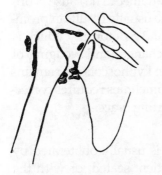

X-ray appearance of a Charcot joint, a possible complication of spinal paralysis

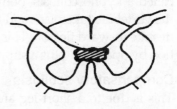

CT appearance of syringomyelia

Scoliosis

Scoliosis of the thoracic and lumbar spine may be fixed or mobile. It may also be compensatory to a short leg or tilted pelvis.

Congenital scoliosis

This is due to a spinal anomaly such as a hemivertebra or other defect and will usually result in a fixed scoliosis which may also be associated with a kyphosis. It may require a spinal support or arthrodesis.

Paralytic scoliosis

This is due to spinal paralysis such as in poliomyelitis, neurofibromatosis or spastic hemiplegia. After a time the scoliosis becomes fixed by ligamentous and bony short-ening and rotation of the vertebrae. It is treated by a sup-porting brace and occasionally by arthrodesis of the spine.

Idiopathic scoliosis

This is usually fixed and is often progressive in child-hood until skeletal maturity is attained. The cause is un-known and rotation of vertebrae usually results in prom-inence of the ribs on one side and a deformity which is called a kyphoscoliosis. Bony changes and wedging of the vertebrae take place and the kyphoscoliosis remains despite forward flexion. This sometimes requires correc-tion by operation plus a supporting brace.

Compensatory scoliosis

This is due to a short leg and is usually obliterated by viewing the back with the patient seated, or with the shortening compensated for by wooden blocks. It is also obliterated by the patient bending forward.

Thoracic and Lumbar Spine Conditions — Scoliosis

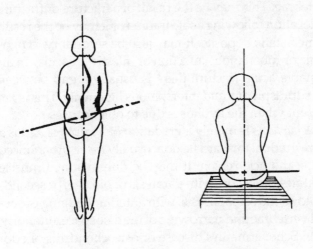

Scoliosis due to leg shortening

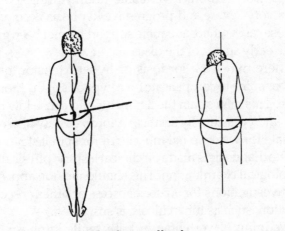

Kyphoscoliosis

Kyphosis and Lordosis

A *kyphos* is a sharp forward flexion deformity of the spine and is usually due to anterior wedging of one or more vertebrae. This may be the result of a fracture or fracture dislocation following acute trauma or it may be the result of metastatic deposits. It may also be secondary to pyogenic or tuberculous infection or infective discitis. In an unstable acute fracture there is usually a gap between the supraspinous and interspinous ligaments. This is *not* present when the kyphos is due to other causes.

A *kyphosis* is merely a gradation of a kyphos, and is a more gradual forward flexion, usually more pronounced in the thoracic region. It may be due to spinal muscle weakness as occurs with paralysis or old age, or secondary to senile osteoporosis, with anterior wedging of several vertebrae and narrowing of the disc space anteriorly.

In Scheuermann's disease or osteochondritis of adolescence there is usually a mild kyphosis due to slight wedging of the thoracic vertebrae. In ankylosing spondylitis a very severe and progressive kyphosis is common in those cases where adequate support has not been given in the early stages of the disease.

There may be a lordosis or hyperextension of the lumbar spine to compensate for a kyphosis in the thoracic spine. This may strain the ligaments and cause low back pain and occasionally sciatica. A lordosis may also compensate for weak spinal muscles or for spinal stenosis.

The diagnosis is made on clinical history, physical and radiological examination. This should include appropriate investigations for a psoas abscess or other abscess if infection, such as tuberculosis, is suspected.

Wedging of vertebrae in both senile kyphosis and Scheuermann's disease can usually be confirmed by

Thoracic and Lumbar Spine Conditions — Kyphosis

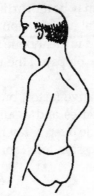

Kyphos

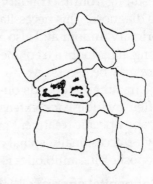

X-ray appearance of a kyphos — secondary to metastatic deposit

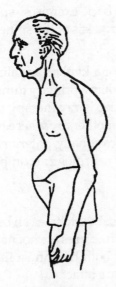

Kyphosis

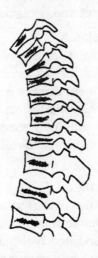

X-ray appearance of senile osteoporotic kyphosis

X-ray, as can a fracture due to trauma. A fracture due to an eosinophilic granuloma (Calvé's disease) usually causes almost complete flattening of a vertebra. Collapse resulting from a secondary deposit may be more difficult to diagnose. This necessitates clinical examination for a primary tumour and also X-rays and nuclear bone scanning. If in doubt a trephine or needle biopsy of the vertebra may be necessary.

Treatment depends on the causative factor, but will often include back extension exercises and a suitable brace. Specific treatment may include deep X-ray therapy or occasionally spinal decompression for secondary deposits plus antibiotics for infection.

Congenital abnormalities

True congenital causes of a kyphosis are due to a defective development of the vertebrae and are uncommon. If symptomatic they may require back exercises, spinal support and occasionally an arthrodesis of the spine.

Neoplasia

Neoplastic causes of a kyphosis or a kyphos are almost always due to a secondary rather than a primary tumour. Treatment usually necessitates deep X-ray therapy plus a back support. Hormones or chemotherapy where indicated may be necessary, and occasionally anterior decompression and stabilisation for neurological compression.

Trauma

Fractures of the thoracic and lumbar vertebrae can be either stable or unstable. The stable fractures are not usually associated with paralysis, and both the infraspinous and the supraspinous ligaments are intact.

Kyphosis — Treatment

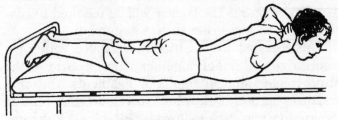

Back exercises

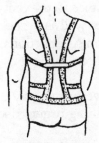

Taylor brace

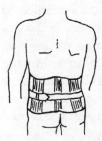

Lumbar support

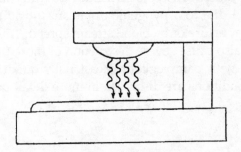

**Deep X-ray therapy
for secondary
deposits**

Treatment is bed rest with back extension braces for about 1–2 weeks. This is followed by support in a lumbar corset which may occasionally extend up to the chest, such as a Taylor brace. The patient will be required to continue with back exercises such as swimming.

Unstable fractures are usually associated with some neurological damage together with rupture of the supraspinous and interspinous ligaments. Unstable fractures in the thoraco-lumbar region may require external stabilisation with rods or cables. Most cases associated with complete transection of the cord are treated conservatively with two hourly turning on a waterbed. Attention to paralysed limbs to prevent contractures and bed sores is essential, as well as sterile catheterisation of the bladder to minimise infections and facilitate an automatic or autonomous bladder (see A Simple Guide to Trauma).

A burst fracture of the lumbar vertebrae may cause pressure on the cauda equina requiring urgent decompression.

Infection

Infective causes of a kyphosis include a discitis (infection of a disc) due to a pyogenic organism introduced by lumbar puncture or by blood stream spread. Tuberculosis may also cause severe destruction of more than one vertebra with paraplegia or occasionally quadriplegia. These conditions are discussed in more detail in Chapter 9.

Kyphosis and Lordosis
Summary of Causes

Neoplasia

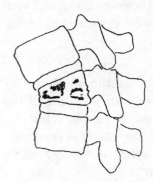 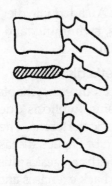

X-ray appearance of a metastatic deposit

X-ray appearance of an eosinophilic granuloma

Trauma

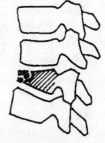 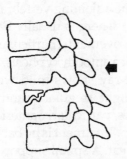

X-ray appearance of a stable vertebral fracture

X-ray appearance of an unstable vertebral fracture

Osteoporotic collapse

This commonly involves several vertebrae, more commonly in the thoracic than the lumbar spine. Back pain and a kyphosis are common, but neurological involvement is rare.

Treatment includes rest plus heat and a spinal support. An adequate diet, with sufficient calcium and vitamins, swimming, and back extension exercises, are essential.

Paget's disease

Paget's disease (chapter 12) may lead to a gradual increasing kyphosis due to the anterior wedging of the thoracic vertebrae. There will usually also be other evidence of Paget's disease. The management is conservative with analgesics plus calcitonin in severe cases together with back exercises and sometimes a back support.

Scheuermann's disease

This condition usually develops in adolescence and affects the bodies of the thoracic and, to a lesser extent, the lumbar vertebrae. It may be due to trauma to the ring epiphyses of the vertebrae with resulting protrusion into the adjoining vertebral bodies.

There is usually back pain with limitation of spinal movements, particularly rotation, with the development of a smooth kyphosis, mainly in the mid thoracic region. X-ray shows mild wedging of several vertebrae with slight irregularity and herniation into the vertebral bodies, particularly anteriorly.

Treatment is by back extension, rotation exercises, and heat. A spinal support may occasionally be indicated.

Kyphosis and Lordosis
Summary of Causes

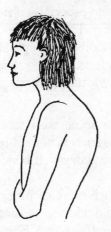

Scheuermann's disease

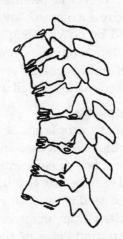

X-ray appearance of Scheuermann's disease

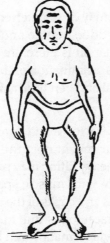

Paget's disease

Back Pain

Congenital abnormalities

Any defect in the integrity of the lumbar spine may progress to chronic low back strain especially if precipitated by heavy lifting and trauma. This includes spina bifida, spondylolysis and spondylolisthesis, spinal stenosis and congenital vertebral defects. These are all discussed in more detail under individual headings.

Neoplasia

Primary neoplasms of the lower spine are uncommon but include soft tissue neoplasms such as neurofibromata and bony neoplasms such as aneurysmal bone cysts and eosinophilic granulomas.

Secondary neoplasms are much more common, particularly from breast, lung, thyroid, kidney, prostate and uterus and these are discussed in Chapter 8. They may involve the sacrum, femora and other bones as well as the lumbar spine.

Pelvic neoplasms may cause referred back pain. These include prostate, bladder, uterine and rectal malignancies. A rectal examination is therefore important where this is indicated, as is examination of the abdomen to exclude gastrointestinal and genitourinary neoplasms.

Trauma

This includes spinal fractures and ligamentous injuries. In many cases recurrent minor trauma, particularly twisting strains and heavy lifting may precipitate an acute episode of 'lumbago' with muscle spasm and referred pain into the buttocks and backs of the thighs. Degenerative changes in the facet joints due to repeated injuries may lead to osteophyte formation and limitation of back

Back Pain
Summary of Causes

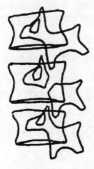

X-ray appearance of spondylolisthesis

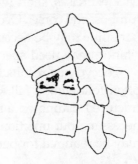

X-ray appearance of vertebral metastases

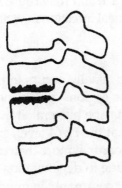

X-ray appearance of spinal infection

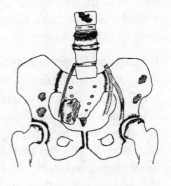

Pelvic causes

movements. Recurrent episodes result in increased stiffness and wasting of muscles.

X-ray may show disc degeneration and osteophyte formation, and treatment is usually conservative with back exercises, short wave diathermy, and sometimes a lumbosacral corset. Occasionally arthrodesis of the lumbar spine may be necessary. Associated sciatic nerve irritation may need specific management (see below).

Coccydynia results from trauma to the coccyx, most often following a fall. Occasionally the coccyx may be fractured. Sitting on a soft cushion is usually all that is necessary, but injection of long acting local anaesthetic may be required for persistent pain.

Infection

Infection of the lumbar spine usually involves a disc space initially. It may occasionally also affect the sacroiliac joint. Infection is discussed further in Chapter 9.

Pelvic infections are common, especially of the bladder, prostate and female genital tract, and may cause referred low back pain. Retroperitoneal infection may also lead to low back pain.

Prolapsed intervertebral disc

Prolapse of an intervertebral disc usually occurs in the L4/5 or L5/S1 intervertebral disc regions and is most often seen on only one side but may be bilateral. It may occur in other regions, especially at the L3/4 level, and occasionally disc protrusion may occur at more than one level simultaneously. It is often due to degeneration of the disc and therefore occurs most commonly in middle or old age.

Degeneration of the annulus fibrosus allows the nucleus pulposus to herniate through a rent in the annulus.

Prolapsed Intervertebral Disc

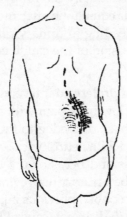

Muscle spasm and compensatory scoliosis

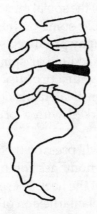

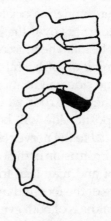

**X-ray appearance of
L4 disc prolapse**

**X-ray appearance of
L5 disc prolapse**

Protrusions at the L4/5 level will thus compress the L5 root, while protrusions at the L5/S1 level will compress the first sacral root. Occasionally the protrusion is central, pressing on the cauda equina and affecting autonomic control of the bladder leading to urinary retention. Urgent surgical decompression of the cauda equina is required as an emergency.

Symptoms and signs of prolapsed intervertebral disc
The classic symptom is low back pain with radiation of severe pain down the back of the leg to the ankle and foot. It may be associated with neurological signs such as motor and sensory loss and occasionally bladder involvement. There may be a history of previous episodes of back pain and sciatica or of a previous injury.

Protrusion of the L4/5 disc may cause L5 root pressure with pain radiating down the leg to the dorsum of the foot. There may be numbness on the outer side of the calf and medial two-thirds of the dorsum of the foot with weakness of dorsiflexion, particularly of the foot and toes. There is often associated spasm of the spinal muscles with tenderness over the lower lumbar spine on the side of the lesion. The muscular spasm may produce a scoliosis. Limitation of lateral flexion of the lumbar spine to the same side will be most marked with a protrusion *lateral* to the nerve root, while limitation of lateral flexion to the opposite side will be most marked with a protrusion *medial* to the nerve root.

Protrusion of the L5/S1 disc will press on the S1 nerve root and may lead to pain and numbness on the outer side of the foot and under side of the heel. There may be weakness of both eversion and plantarflexion of the foot with a diminished or absent knee jerk.

Prolapsed Intervertebral Disc

Sensory and motor deficit

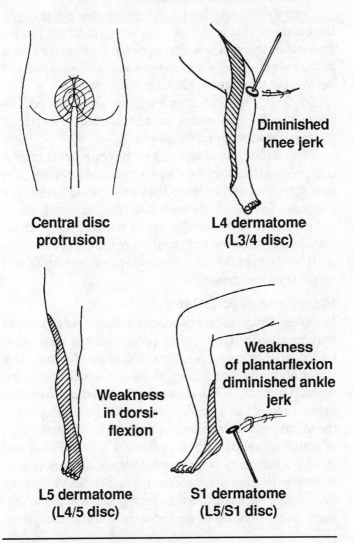

Central disc protrusion

Diminished knee jerk

L4 dermatome (L3/4 disc)

Weakness in dorsiflexion

L5 dermatome (L4/5 disc)

Weakness of plantarflexion diminished ankle jerk

S1 dermatome (L5/S1 disc)

Protrusion of the L3/4 disc may cause pressure on the L4 nerve root and may lead to numbness over the front of the knee and leg with diminution of the knee jerk and weakness of the knee extensors.

Central protrusion of a lower lumbar disc can press on the cauda equina and lead to urinary retention. On examination there is usually perianal numbness and a patulous anus. *Emergency decompression is essential* to avoid permanent damage to sphincter innervation.

Disc protrusions at other levels are less common. Occasionally pressure on the cord itself at a higher level may cause paraplegia, or quadriplegia.

The differential diagnosis of lumbar neurological compression includes the various causes of low back pain (see above) as well as the causes of localised nerve root pressure. These include secondary tumours and multiple myeloma of the lumbar spine which usually cause vertebral destruction with sparing of the discs. Fractures and infections of the spine may also cause nerve root and spinal cord compression.

Miscellaneous conditions

Pathology involving thoracic abdominal or pelvic viscera may produce referred spinal pain, which at times may be the first, or even only, sign of disease. Thoracic and upper abdominal pathology tends to produce pain in the thoraco-lumbar legion, lower abdominal diseases in the lumbar region, and pelvic diseases tend to refer pain to the sacral region. On examination there are often no signs of actual spinal pathology ie. there is little stiffness and there is a full range of movement. Peptic ulceration, gastroduodenal tumours, pancreatitis and cholecystitis may all produce back pain, as may retroperitoneal pathology such as lymphomas or an abdominal aortic aneurysm.

Back Pain

Summary of Causes
in the lumbar spine and pelvis

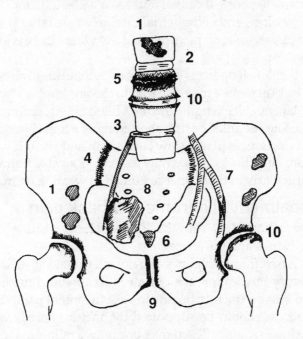

1. Secondary deposits
2. Low back strain
3. Prolapsed disc
4. Ankylosing spondylitis
5. Trauma
6. Coccydynia
7. Vascular
8. Pelvic tumour
9. Gynaecological
10. Osteoarthritis

Lumbar back pain may result from colonic conditions such as colitis, diverticulitis or colo-rectal neoplasms. Sacral pain is usually a result of urologic or gynaecological diseases. Uterine malposition (eg. retroversion) and dysmenorrhoea may produce sacral pain, but the latter is usually poorly localised and has a wide radiation. Endometriosis and endometrial carcinoma are other possible causes of sacral pain, particularly where there is local invasion.

Senile osteoporosis or poor muscle tone due to obesity or lack of exercise may also lead to chronic low back pain.

Unequal leg lengths due to a tilted pelvis, deformed hip, knee or ankle or true shortening of a leg will also, if left uncorrected, cause low back strain and chronic back pain. High heeled shoes may also cause low back strain, particularly in those unaccustomed to wearing them.

Treatment of chronic low back pain

The management of low back pain includes treating both the causes and the effects.

Apart from analgesics and non-steroidal anti-inflammatory medication, the optimum treatment consists of bed rest on fracture boards to ease the initial pain. The mattress should be supported by fracture boards with the knees slightly flexed over one or two pillows. This is followed by an exercise program to strengthen the back muscles together with heat. Education regarding sitting, lying and lifting is essential and swimming is the most effective long term exercise. Occasionally a lumbosacral corset, worn while the patient is working or travelling, will help relieve the pain. Pain relief is best achieved by mobilising the spine and strengthening the back muscles. Manipulation under anaesthesia may also be indicated in chronic cases *without* sciatic compression.

Back Pain — Treatment

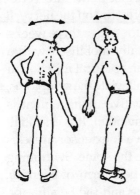

Physiotherapy

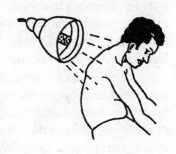

Heat

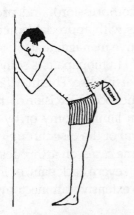

Local anaesthetic spray and extension exercises

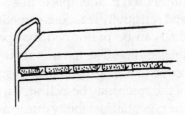

Fracture boards

In the case of sciatic irritation due to a prolapsed disc, skin traction of about three to four kilograms on each leg, or alternatively, pelvic traction, will help to distract the lumbar vertebrae and increase the size of the intervertebral foramina, thus relieving the pressure on the nerve. It may be necessary to continue this for two or three weeks, and the patient should be gradually mobilised with a lumbosacral brace. Occasionally an epidural injection of local anaesthetic and steroids will alleviate the symptoms.

In over 90% of cases, conservative management is successful and operation can be avoided. It is essential, however, that patients build up weak extensor muscles of the spine and regularly exercise the spine. Swimming in a warm pool is probably the best form of exercise. Education regarding lifting, sitting and the benefit of a regular exercise program is also essential (Chapter 6).

Although most cases will respond to conservative measures, the indications for operation include cauda equina lesions (emergency decompression), and progressive or unresponsive lesions with appreciable neurological signs despite conservative management.

In acute lesions, injections of chymopapain is sometimes used in attempts to dissolve the disc. This may fail and sensitivity reactions sometimes occur. Excision of the disc can be performed by open laminectomy or by a nucleotome. The latter is removal of the disc through a scope like an arthroscope. In some cases, an arthrodesis of the spine may be indicated for severe back pain, or for the potential instability due to an extensive laminectomy.

Back Pain — Treatment

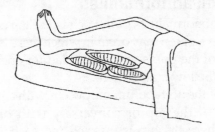

Bed rest and supports

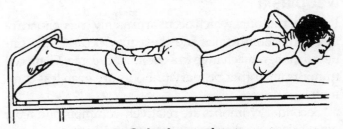

Spinal exercises

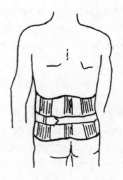

Lumbar corset

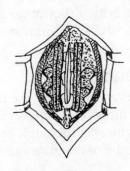

Laminectomy or arthrodesis

Pelvic and Sacral Conditions

Congenital abnormalities

Congenital abnormalities of the pelvis itself are uncommon but an ectropion may occur in which there is a defect in the front of the pubis so that the bladder opens on to the front of the lower abdomen.

Defects of the acetabulum may occur with congenital dislocation of the hip or conversely with protrusio acetabuli where the hip is inserted more deeply than normal into the pelvis.

Neoplasia

Primary tumours which occur are mainly osteochondromas or enchondromas and these may occasionally undergo malignant change to a chondrosarcoma. Giant cell tumours and other primary tumours are even less common.

Secondary tumours are relatively common, and have often arisen from primary tumours in the breast, lung, thyroid, kidney, prostate or uterus. Such tumours are usually treated conservatively with deep X-ray therapy, together with hormones or chemotherapy if appropriate. Almost all other primary tumours can result in secondary spread to the pelvis.

Trauma

Fractures of pelvis are common. Shear (vertical force) fractures may be associated with sciatic nerve palsy. Fractures of the pubic ramus may cause rupture of the bladder or membranous urethra.

Pelvic and Sacral Conditions

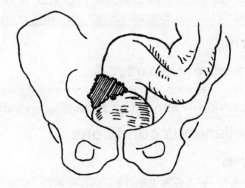

**Carcinoma involving
bladder and rectum**

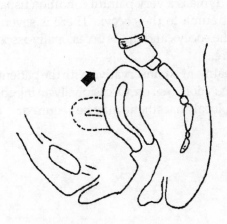

Retroflexed uterus

Infection

Pyogenic arthritis of the hip occurs mainly following internal fixation of hip fractures or hip replacements. Infections of the sacroiliac joint by pyogenic organisms or Mycobacterium tuberculosis are very uncommon.

Arthritis

Degenerative (osteoarthritis)

There may be secondary degenerative osteoarthritis in joints previously affected by ankylosing spondylitis.

Miscellaneous conditions

Paralysis

In poliomyelitis and some other paralytic conditions in childhood, such as meningomyelocele, the pelvis on one or both sides may be small or poorly developed.

Coccydynia

Coccydynia is a very painful condition usually resulting from trauma to the coccyx. There is severe tenderness over the coccyx and this is occasionally associated with a fracture.

Treatment is conservative with the patient using a soft foam cushion to sit on. Occasionally an injection of a long-acting local anaesthetic may be required.

Pelvic and Sacral Conditions

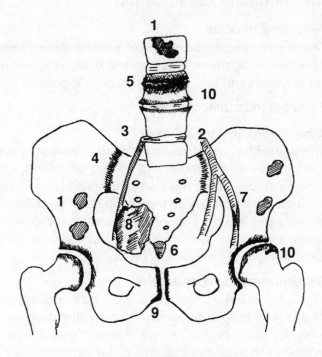

1. Secondary deposits
2. Low back strain
3. Prolapsed disc
4. Ankylosing spondylitis
5. Trauma
6. Coccydynia
7. Vascular
8. Pelvic tumour
9. Gynaecological
10. Osteoarthritis

Peripheral Nerve Lesions

Aetiological Classification

Peripheral neuritis

The many causes include diabetes, alcoholism and toxicity. There is usually sensory loss and burning sensation of the fingers and toes with normal muscle power.

Peroneal muscular atrophy

(Charcot–Marie–Tooth disease)

This is an autosomal dominant condition often first presenting in early childhood and leading to clawing and wasting of the intrinsic muscles of the hands and feet.

There may be a pes cavus, weakness of the peroneal muscles and loss of proprioceptive sensation below the knees. Foot supports, calipers and occasionally operative correction of deformities may be required.

Duchenne muscular dystrophy

This has a sex linked recessive pattern of inheritance, and thus is seen only in males. It is usually first diagnosed when the child begins to walk. There is pseudohypertrophy of the calf muscles due to fat deposition. Progressive weakness usually means that the child is unable to walk by age 10 and will commonly die by the age of 20. Splinting and tendon transfers may help.

Friedreich's ataxia

This is an inherited disorder with progressive degeneration of the posterolateral columns of the spinal cord and part of the cerebellum. The child has an ataxic gait as well as clawing and varus deformity of the feet.

Peripheral Nerve Lesions

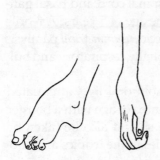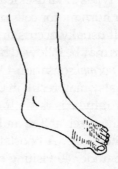

Charcot–Marie–Tooth disease   **Peripheral neuritis**

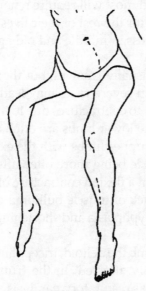

Poliomyelitis

Poliomyelitis

Poliomyelitis is a paralytic condition caused by one of three types of viruses leading to the disruption of the anterior horn motor cells of the spinal cord and basal ganglia. It usually occurs under the age of 5 years. A febrile illness may be followed by a flaccid, *asymmetrical* paralysis with *normal* sensation. Occasionally respiratory and bulbar palsy may result in death.

Prophylaxis is with the Sabin oral live, attenuated vaccine given at 2, 4, and 6 months of age with a booster at school age. A booster dose should also be taken by those under 40 visiting countries in the tropics and subtropics where large epidemics are still occurring in the 1990s. In these countries there are still many millions of untreated paralytic patients. In economically developed countries most polio patients were paralysed 30–40 years ago in infancy and most will require renewal of calipers and other splints for the rest of their lives. Occasionally increasing weakness in middle and old age will require further treatment.

Bulbar palsy usually resolves, but the asymmetrical flaccid paralysis in severe cases may lead not only to a flail limb, but also to contractures due to the unbalanced muscle action. The lower limbs are often more severely affected than the upper limbs with the extensors of the hip, knee and ankle being more often affected than the flexors resulting in a flexion contracture of the hip, knee and ankle. The lack of muscle bulk in a growing child will also lead to hypoplasia and shortening of the affected limb.

In the upper limb the deltoid, triceps and thenar muscles are commonly affected. In the trunk, scoliosis is common as well as respiratory paralysis.

Poliomyelitis

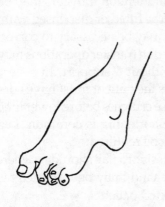

Pes cavus and toe clawing

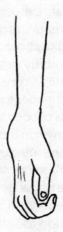

Clawing of hands

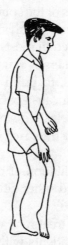

Wasted, contracted, hip, knee and ankle

Recovery will only occur in the first few months of paralysis and residual paralysis of the lower limbs may necessitate calipers to enable the patient to walk.

Soft tissue fasciotomies and tendon transfers may be required to allow a caliper to be fitted or dispensed with. An osteotomy or arthodesis may be necessary to correct a deformity. Appropriate tendon transfer operations may enable a patient to walk without a support. In severe paralysis of both lower limbs the patient must have adequate power in the arms to use crutches before lower limb operations are performed. Shortening is common. Leg equalisation operations may be required.

In the upper limb arthrodesis of a flail shoulder, where the patient has a functional hand, may be indicated, as will tendon transfers in selected patients.

A very weak trunk with scoliosis may require a supporting corset to enable a patient to sit unsupported. Extensive arthrodesis of the spine may prevent a patient with severe lower limb paralysis walking with calipers and should be avoided in most cases.

Intensive physiotherapy is usually needed to prevent muscle contractures, to build up partially paralysed muscles and to re-educate a patient in walking.

Complications include dislocations of a hip due to weak abductors and fractures of the thin osteoporotic bones.

The social rehabilitation of the patient is important, with wheelchairs and other aids for the severely paralysed.

The principles of treatment of polio patients will often apply to other patients with paralysis due to spina bifida, fractures, strokes.

Poliomyelitis — Treatment

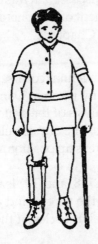

Polio patient with caliper and stick

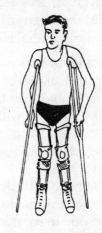

Polio patient with calipers and crutches

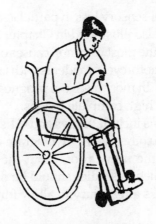

Polio patient in a wheelchair

Anatomical classification — upper limb

Individual nerve lesions will be discussed in this chapter whilst the diagnosis and assessment of peripheral nerve lesions in general is discussed in Chapter 2.

Brachial plexus

The brachial plexus extends from spinal cord segments C5 to T1 and may be damaged by trauma. Damage to roots C5 and C6 will lead to paralysis of the deltoid and external rotators of the shoulders. The arm is held in internal rotation and extension (waiter's tip position, or Erb's palsy).

Damage to the lower roots (C7, 8, and T1) leads to a flexed elbow due to paralysis of the triceps and a weak hand due to paralysis of the small muscles of the hand (T1 innervation).

A complete brachial plexus lesion will lead to a flail, wasted arm held in extension and internally rotated with complete sensory loss.

The extent of sensory loss in partial lesions of the brachial plexus is also illustrated in Chapter 2.

In adult life the most common causes of brachial plexus injuries are motorcycle accidents with falls on the point of the shoulder. In most cases the prognosis is very poor, especially with high complete lesions.

Investigations include X-rays and CT scans of the cervical spine and sometimes a myelogram or MRI scan to show tears of the nerve roots from the cervical cord. Electrical conduction studies should be delayed until at least three weeks after injury to allow for settling of the spinal shock.

Treatment initially consists of relaxing the brachial plexus with a splint in about 60° of abduction. Steroids may also be given to reduce oedema of the nerve roots.

Upper Limb Nerve Lesions

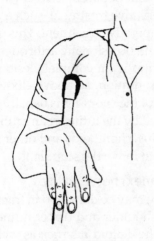

Radial nerve palsy

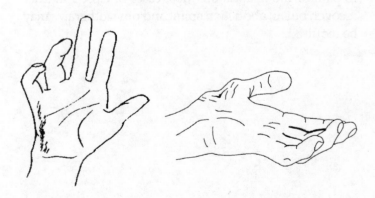

Ulnar nerve palsy   **Median nerve palsy**

There may also be an indication for operative exploration and repair of a postaxonal (low) lesion, but this is often very difficult and the prognosis poor.

Late management of partial lesions which do not recover with conservative treatment, such as physiotherapy, may require operative treatment. This usually entails tendon transfer and occasionally arthrodesis of the wrist or the use of supports. In complete lesions with a flail arm and absent sensation, an above elbow amputation with arthrodesis of the shoulder is usually the treatment of choice, followed by the fitting of an artificial arm, provided the trapezius, rhomboids and other muscles have adequate power to move the scapula.

Axillary (circumflex) nerve palsy

The axillary nerve may be damaged in fractures and dislocations of the shoulder and upper humerus. There is numbness over the deltoid *insertion* as well as paralysis of the deltoid. The inability of the patient to abduct the arm may be due to paralysis of the deltoid or merely due to pain or the dislocation. Most cases of closed injuries recover, but an abduction splint and physiotherapy may be required.

Brachial Plexus Lesions

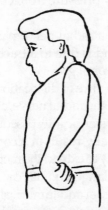

**Erb's palsy showing
'waiter's tip' position**

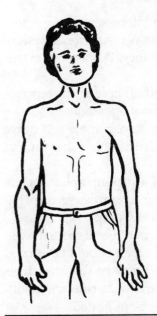

Diagnosis

1. Altered nerve response
   to electrical stimulation
2. Absent or diminished
   sensation and sweating
3. Flail or weak arm

Radial nerve lesion

A high radial nerve palsy may be due to pressure on the nerve in the axilla by pressure from crutches that are too long.

The usual site of a radial nerve palsy, is however, in the mid humerus and is due to a fracture with pressure on the nerve in the spiral groove.

Occasionally a fracture or dislocation at the elbow may cause a low lesion of the radial nerve, affecting mainly its distal branch, the posterior interosseous nerve.

High lesions usually result in a complete wrist drop together with inability to extend the metacarpophalangeal joints. The interphalangeal joints can, however, be extended by the interossei and lumbricals (supplied by the ulnar and median nerves). There is also associated numbness over the base of the thumb and the back of the hand.

Low lesions of the posterior interosseus nerve below the long extensors of the wrist may result in paralysis of extensors of the metacarpophalangeal joints with extension of the wrist intact.

Most closed lesions of the radial nerve are incomplete and over 80% will recover without operation.

Investigations include electromyographic and nerve conduction studies, but these are of little value until at least 3 weeks after the injury.

Initial treatment consists of a cock-up splint for the wrist combined with springs to maintain extension of the metacarpophalangeal joints (lively splint).

If a complete division of the nerve is suspected early exploration and microsurgical repair should be carried out. Occasionally nerve grafting may be required. If recovery does not occur tendon transfers, combined with an arthrodesis of the wrist, may be indicated.

Radial Nerve Lesion

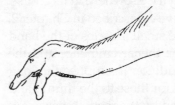
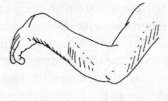

Low level nerve injury   **High level nerve injury**

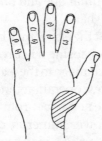

Sensory deficit

Treatment

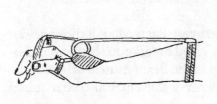
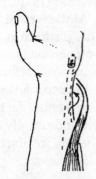

Splint   **Arthrodesis and tendon transfer**

Ulnar nerve lesion

The ulnar nerve is injured commonly at the elbow. It may, however, sustain an open injury elsewhere in its course. Examination of the ulnar nerve is described in Chapter 2.

The nerve supplies all the small muscles of the hand except for the muscles of the thenar eminence and the lateral two lumbricals. In addition it supplies the long flexors of the fingers, except for those to the thumb and forefinger which are supplied by the median nerve but there is often an overlap. The ulnar nerve also supplies the sensation to the ulnar one and one half fingers and to the ulnar side of the hand.

The ulnar nerve at the elbow may be damaged by blunt trauma to the elbow causing a neuropraxia (concussion) or an axonotmesis (damage to the axon continuity). Fractures round the elbow, operations and open injuries may completely sever the nerve (neurotmesis). In addition an old fracture of the lower humerus, particularly a supracondylar fracture in a child, may cause epiphyseal damage with an increasing valgus deformity of the elbow. This can lead to a late (tardy) nerve palsy due to gradual stretching of the nerve over the medial condyle.

At the wrist a fracture on the ulnar side of the lower ulna, pisiform or hamate may cause nerve damage or compression, as may a synovitis in conditions such as rheumatoid arthritis.

In open injuries microvascular repair is indicated. The nerve should be transferred anterior to the medial condyle and usually deep to the flexor muscle origin. Neurolysis or freeing of the nerve alone may also be required in late palsy.

Ulnar Nerve Lesion

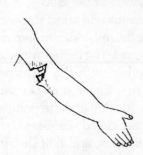

Compound fracture above the elbow

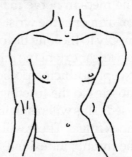

Old supracondylar fracture

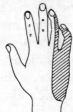

Dorsum

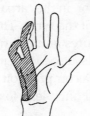

Palm

Sensory deficit

Treatment

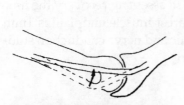

Anterior transfer of nerve at the elbow

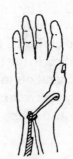

Tendon transfer

Median nerve lesion

The median nerve may be divided at the elbow, in the forearm or at the wrist. High lesions will affect the nerve supply to the long flexors of the thumb, index finger, and to a lesser extent the middle fingers. The thenar muscles, except adductor pollicis, together with the lumbrical muscles to the forefinger and ring finger, are also paralysed. This will result in a loss of flexion and the pointing index finger. There will also be associated numbness over the thumb, index and middle fingers, and half the ring finger together with two-thirds of the palm.

Median nerve compression at the wrist may occur due to compression in the carpal tunnel when it is narrowed in the front of the wrist. This narrowing may occur not only in fractures and arthritis of the wrist, but also following soft tissue oedema in rheumatoid arthritis and in pregnancy. Decompression by division of the flexor retinaculum will often lead to a dramatic and complete recovery.

Repair of a divided median nerve is best carried out by microsurgical techniques except where there is a dirty wound, in which case wound healing should first be achieved. There is occasionally a place for replacing a nerve defect by cable grafting from a cutaneous nerve. In cases where recovery does not occur, tendon transfers may be indicated to restore flexion of the forefinger and opposition to the thumb. In assessing recovery the time of regeneration to the nearest muscle endplate is 1mm per day. Electromyographic and nerve conduction studies can also assess recovery.

Median Nerve Lesion

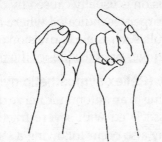

Testing for motor weakness

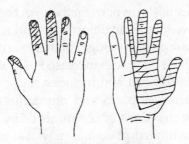

Dorsum   **Palm**

Sensory deficit

Treatment

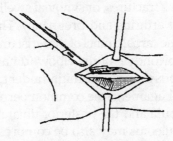

Exploration and microsurgical repair

Digital nerve division

Digital nerve division is usually caused by direct injury. Suture by microsurgery is indicated where a significant disability will result, such as nerve division on the radial side of the index finger or both sides of the thumb.

Sudek's atrophy (Reflex sympathetic dystrophy)

This is probably due to an autonomic nerve dysfunction, and is usually associated with severe fractures of the upper limb. It may also occur following a stroke or myocardial infarction.

The patient will often have trophic skin changes and severe hyperaesthesia (hypersensitivity) of the skin. Discolouration, sweating, joint deformities and stiffness are common. Radiological investigation may show marked osteoporosis and a bone scan increased vascularity.

Treatment is difficult and includes supports to prevent contractures, ice packs and physiotherapy. Sympathectomy by injections of chemicals or by operative division have a limited place and may also cause complications.

Nerve entrapment

Bone or soft tissue may press on nerves where they traverse fibro-osseous sheaths. This may be due to overuse, to previous fractures, or synovial swelling as occurs in rheumatoid arthritis and pregnancy. The most common sites are the carpal tunnel of the wrist (median nerve), and medial epicondyle of the elbow (ulnar nerve). The lateral cutaneous nerve of the thigh under the lateral end of the inguinal ligament, the common peroneal nerve at the neck of fibula and the posterior tibial nerve behind the medial malleolus may also be compressed. Decompression may lead to rapid relief of symptoms.

Other Nerve Injuries

Digital nerve

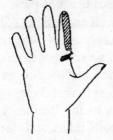

Laceration causing digital
nerve damage

Nerve entrapment

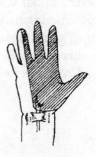

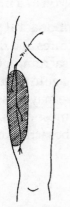

Median nerve
entrapment in carpal
tunnel syndrome

Lateral cutaneous
nerve of thigh

Anatomical classification — lower limb

Cauda equina

Damage to the cauda equina is often a surgical emergency as it usually causes bladder paralysis with retention or incontinence as well as weakness of the lower limbs.

The most common cause of paralysis is damage from a fracture of the lumbar spine or from central prolapse of an intervertebral disc. Damage, however, may also occur in spondylolisthesis, spina bifida, or as a complication of secondary deposits in the lumbar vertebrae. Neurofibromatosis and spinal infections may also cause paralysis.

The diagnosis is on clinical grounds and one or more of the following may be present: perianal numbness, a patulous anus, variable degrees of paralysis and urinary retention. Investigations should include a CT or MRI scan as well as X-rays.

Treatment may involve a laminectomy and decompression as a matter of *urgency* in most cases.

Lumbosacral plexus

Fractures and dislocation of the lower lumbar vertebrae and sacrum, or the posterior part of the pelvis, may cause damage to the lower lumbar and upper sacral nerve roots. These may occasionally require operative decompression, but most cases are treated with bed rest followed by a lumbosacral support.

Cauda Equina Lesions

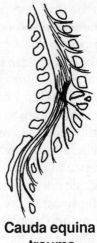

Cauda equina trauma

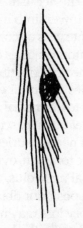

Neoplasm of cauda equina

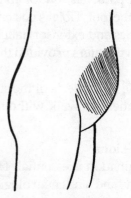

Bladder paralysis

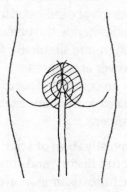

Sensory loss

Sciatic nerve lesions

Examination for partial or complete sciatic nerve compression is discussed above in prolapsed intervertebral disc. The nerve may also be damaged in pelvic fractures, or in lower limb injuries. Damage to the common peroneal nerve is often seen with dislocations and severe ligamentous injuries of the knee and upper fibula.

The posterior tibial nerve may also be damaged in knee injuries and can be trapped under the retinaculum posterior to the medial malleolus, especially in ankle fractures.

Treatment of sciatic, posterior tibial and common peroneal nerve injuries varies from neurolysis at the greater sciatic foramen, over the neck of the fibula, or behind the medial malleolus, to microsurgical repair.

In posterior tibial and complete sciatic nerve injuries, sensory loss may necessitate special footwear to prevent sores under the heel. Foot drop may require a caliper or splint to support the foot with the addition of a toe raising spring.

In certain cases of incomplete paralysis, tendon transfers may be indicated to balance the foot. Tibialis posterior and anterior, the peroneal muscles and extensor hallucis longus are all suitable for tendon transfers provided their power is at least 4.

In complete foot drop a triple arthrodesis of the subtaloid joints may enable the patient to walk without a caliper.

Investigation of sciatic nerve lesions

A full history and clinical examination is essential. This includes examination of the spine and a full neurological assessment, together with a full examination of the rest of the patient, including an abdominal and a rectal examination. Carcinoma of the prostate, bladder, uterus or

Investigation of Sciatica

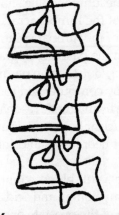

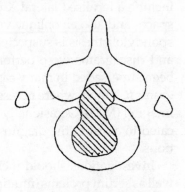

X-ray appearance of spondylolisthesis

CT scan appearance of a prolapsed disc

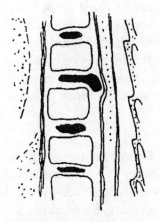

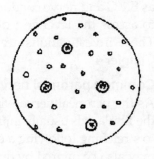

MRI scan appearance of a prolapsed disc

Haematological investigations

rectum are relatively common causes of low back pain and sciatica.

Radiological examination of the lumbar spine should include a localised lateral X-ray of the lumbosacral disc spaces and also an oblique view of the lumbar spine if a spondylolisthesis is suspected. In the past, myelograms and discograms were performed, but these have now been superseded in many cases by computerised tomograms (CT) and, where necessary, by magnetic resonance imaging (MRI). Occasionally a nuclear bone scan is indicated to assist in the diagnosis of neoplasms and infections.

Investigations should include a full blood count, as well as serum proteins (multiple myeloma), and acid and alkaline phosphatase (carcinoma of the prostate or multiple secondaries respectively), where indicated.

Serum agglutinins for salmonella and brucella may occasionally be indicated. Other investigations may include urine analysis and X-rays of chest or pelvis if tuberculosis is suspected, or if there is a possibility of secondary deposits. Very occasionally electrical studies such as EMG and nerve conduction studies may be indicated to assess the level and degree of nerve compressions. These investigations are described in more detail in Chapter 4.

Common peroneal nerve

As the peroneal nerve winds around the upper part of the fibula, it is usually injured either by a fracture or due to stretching following a dislocation of the knee joint. It may also be injured by direct pressure, for example, if a plaster cast is too tight and occasionally by direct pressure over the nerve following unsatisfactory positioning on the operating table.

Lower Limb Nerve Lesions

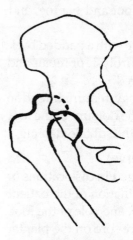

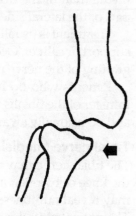

X-ray appearance of a posterior dislocation of the hip

X-ray appearance of a dislocated knee

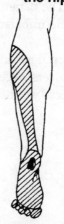

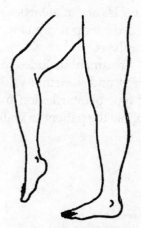

Tibial nerve palsy

Common peroneal nerve palsy

The patient usually has a complete foot drop in complete nerve lesions, together with numbness over the medial half of the dorsum of the foot and big toe, and part of the lateral side of the calf.

Treatment is usually conservative with a padded back support or caliper. Occasionally neurolysis or repair and grafting of the nerve may be required.

Patients who do not recover may require a tendon transfer of the tibialis posterior to the dorsum of the foot and occasionally an arthrodesis of the subtaloid joints.

Tibial nerve (medial popliteal nerve)

The tibial nerve may also be damaged in dislocations of the knee or by open injuries. Examination of the patient may reveal numbness over the heel and sole of the foot. The patient may develop a pressure sore on the plantar surface of the foot as a result of absent or impaired sensation.

There is either partial or complete paralysis of the calf muscles and plantarflexion of the toes. The patient may also develop a cavus foot due to muscle imbalance or paralysis.

Treatment includes soft footwear to prevent pressure areas, and sometimes skin grafting for ulcers. Weakness of foot plantarflexion may require special splinting to enable the patient to walk.

Chapter 12

Metabolic and Endocrine Bone Disease

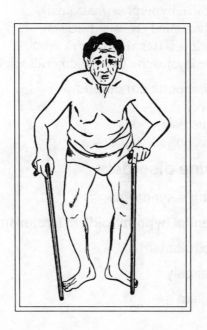

Classification

Metabolic disorders

Osteoporosis

Paget's disease

Hyperparathyroidism

Osteomalacia and Rickets
Osteomalacia
Nutritional rickets
Coeliac or gluten-induced rickets
Familial hyperphosphataemia
(vitamin D resistant rickets)
Cystinosis (renal tubular rickets)
Osteodystrophy (renal glomerular rickets)

Miscellaneous conditions
Scurvy
Industrial poisons
Mucopolysaccharidoses

Endocrine disorders

Cushing's syndrome

Congenital hypothyroidism (cretinism)

Hypopituitarism

Acromegaly

Gigantism

Metabolic and Endocrine Bone Disease

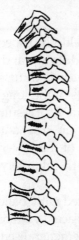

X-ray appearance of osteoporosis

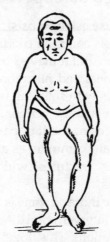

Paget's disease

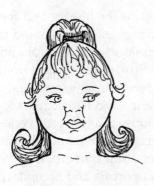

Facial appearance in Cushing's syndrome

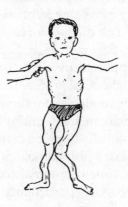

Rickets

Metabolic Disorders

Senile osteoporosis

(Diffuse osteoporosis)

This is a common condition in the elderly, especially in women, but it may also occur in middle age and have a hormonal and nutritional basis. There is diffuse osteoporosis with thinning of the cortices of the long bones, particularly the vertebrae and femora. As a result of this, fractures of the hip, particularly in the trochanteric region, are common, as are fractures of the lower radius (Colles' fractures) which occur with relatively minor trauma.

The thoracic spine is often involved with 'ballooning' of the intervertebral discs into the adjacent vertebrae (see illustration). This, together with the generalised osteoporosis, often causes wedging of the vertebrae following minor, or unrecognised, trauma thus producing a gradually increasing kyphosis.

The diagnosis relies mainly on the history and the classical radiological appearance of osteoporosis and is supported by a relatively normal haematological and biochemical profile. This will help to differentiate it from osteomalacia, parathyroid osteodystrophy, secondary carcinomatosis, multiple myeloma and leukaemia. Occasionally trephine or needle biopsy of a collapsed vertebra or a histopathological examination of tissue taken at the time of internal fixation of a hip fracture, may be necessary, particularly as osteoporosis and secondary carcinomatosis may co-exist.

The general treatment of the patient should include an adequate exercise programme, especially swimming if possible. Good nutrition is also very important,

Metabolic Disorders

Senile Osteoporosis

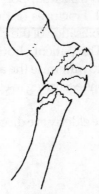

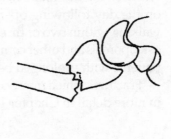

X-ray appearance of an intertrochanteric fracture

X-ray appearance of a Colles' fracture

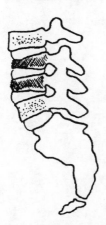

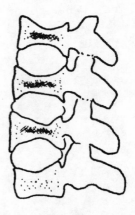

X-ray appearance of a crush fracture with wedging

X-ray appearance of disc 'ballooning'

including multivitamins and minerals (especially a high calcium diet) as many elderly people have a deficient diet and very little exercise.

Physiotherapy, heat, and possibly a back support worn during the day, may be beneficial. Fractures of the hip will need internal fixation, with mobilisation of the patient on the day following operation. The patient should be walking within two or three days to minimise the added osteoporosis and other complications occurring in elderly patients with prolonged bed rest.

Fractures which may occur in the elderly are discussed in more detail in Chapter 15.

Senile Osteoporosis — Treatment

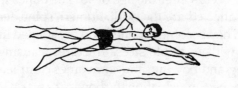

Exercise

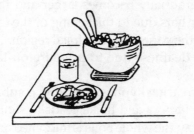

Nutrition

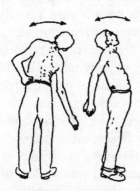

Physiotherapy

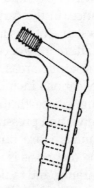

Internal fixation of fractures

Paget's disease

Paget's disease may affect one or many bones. The cause is unknown but is probably due to a viral infection. It usually occurs after the age of 40. The bones most commonly affected are the skull, humeri, spine, femora and tibiae. They become softened and broadened in the early stages with multiple stress fractures, causing gradual bending and bowing, and sometimes complete fracture of the bone. On palpation the bones are warm, thickened and slightly tender.

The skull gradually becomes larger and the patient requires larger hats due to thickening of the calvarium, particularly in the parietal and occipital region. There may be increasing deafness due to pressure on the eighth cranial nerve.

There is increasing kyphosis and this, combined with bowing of the femora and tibiae, leads to shortening of stature. On X-ray, the whole bone is thickened and bowed with loss of distinction between cortex and medulla. There is widening of the cortex, coarsening of the bony trabeculae with cystic and sclerotic areas giving a spongy appearance. In the early stages the bone is very vascular and because of this high pulse pressure high output cardiac failure may occur. Later this vascularity is replaced with sclerotic areas which may be very hard. Possible complications include multiple fractures with delayed healing, osteoarthritis of the hip and knee, deformity of the pelvis and pressure on the spinal nerves. Osteogenic sarcoma is a rare, but invariably fatal complication.

The diagnosis is usually made on the classical X-ray appearance, and radio-isotope scanning shows markedly increased uptake in the affected bones. The alkaline

Metabolic Disorders

Paget's Disease

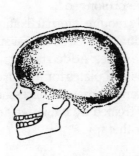

X-ray appearance of a thickened calvarium

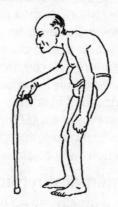

Kyphosis

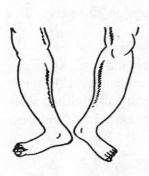

Bowing of the tibia and femur

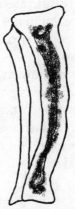

X-ray appearance of tibial thickening and bowing

phosphatase level is usually high and the urinary hydroxyproline level is elevated.

In many cases, no treatment is required and despite the severe deformities, there is often only minimal pain. If pain is severe, however, intravenous calcitonin or oral biphosphonates may provide relief, as they reduce bone turnover, but treatment must be prolonged.

Pathological fractures usually require internal fixation, as non-union is common. Bleeding may be severe at surgery, especially in the more acute stages. Added bone graft is important in addition to nails and plates for fractures. Occasionally a total hip replacement may be necessary. Osteogenic sarcoma is usually treated by palliative amputation and occasionally radiotherapy.

Hyperparathyroidism

This is usually caused by an adenoma of the parathyroid glands and can also occur in renal failure. The bones become thin with multiple cystic areas (osteitis fibrosa cystica) due to absorption of calcium from the bones and its excretion in the urine. This may lead to pathological fractures, renal calculi or indigestion and generalised weakness.

X-rays show multiple cystic areas in the long bones, the skull shows granular mottling and cystic areas, and there may be cortical erosion in the phalanges. The serum calcium is increased and phosphate diminished while urinary excretion of both is increased. Treatment is the removal of the tumour.

Metabolic Disorders

Paget's Disease

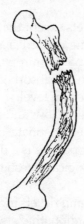

X-ray appearance of a pathological fracture

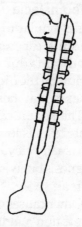

X-ray appearance of internal fixation

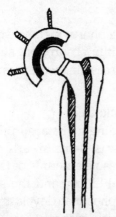

X-ray appearance of a total hip replacement

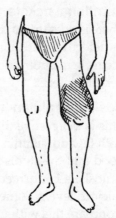

Osteogenic sarcoma

Osteomalacia and rickets

Rickets is defective calcification in growing bone whilst osteomalacia is the same condition in adults, after the epiphyseal plates have fused.

Osteomalacia

This is similar to nutritional rickets except that it occurs in adults, especially in developing countries and in the elderly. It is due to a deficiency of vitamin D and often calcium in the diet so that calcium is reabsorbed from the bones to maintain an adequate serum level.

The serum calcium is normal or low and the phosphate level is low, whilst alkaline phosphatase readings are usually elevated. Senile osteoporosis is a differential diagnosis but with this, haematological investigations are normal.

Other causes of osteomalacia and rickets include malabsorption syndromes such as idiopathic steatorrhoea where there is deficient absorption of fats, fat soluble vitamin D and calcium.

Nutritional rickets

There is a disturbed calcium-phosphorus metabolism due to defective nutrition and calcium absorption, such as occurs in malnutrition, coeliac disease and various familial genetic defects.

Coeliac or gluten-induced rickets

This is a digestive disorder leading to malabsorption of both fat and vitamin D. The disease starts in early childhood and the stools show excessive amounts of fat. Diagnosis is confirmed by jejunal biopsy and the serum calcium levels. Sometimes the phosphate levels are low (compare this with nutritional rickets above).

Metabolic Disorders

Osteomalacia and rickets

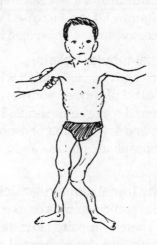

Child with rickets

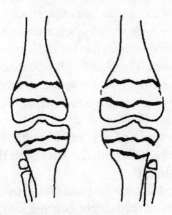

**X-ray appearance of
widened epiphyses**

Familial hyperphosphataemia (vitamin D resistant)

This is a hereditary disorder due to an X-linked gene. It is probably due to a failure of reabsorption of phosphate by the renal tubules or the intestine. There is usually a normal serum calcium and a low serum phosphate (not corrected by vitamin D), an increased alkaline phosphatase and excessive loss of phosphate in the urine.

Cystinosis (renal tubular rickets)

This is due to a recessive genetic defect which results in a failure of the renal tubules to reabsorb not only phosphate but also glucose and some amino acids. There is normal plasma calcium and low plasma phosphate whilst urinary levels of phosphate, glucose and amino acids are increased.

Osteodystrophy (renal glomerular rickets)

This is due to a chronic nephritis or to congenital polycystic kidneys. There is impaired excretion of phosphorus by the kidneys and this is excreted in the intestine where it binds with calcium to form insoluble calcium phosphate which cannot be reabsorbed.

Skeletal changes usually occur between the ages of 5 and 10. The child is deformed and dwarfed with signs of renal impairment. The plasma phosphate is increased and the plasma calcium low. There are signs of renal failure including a high blood urea and serum creatinine as well as albuminuria.

In all these types of rickets, although the biochemical changes may be different, the effects on the patient and skeleton are similar.

The general health and skeletal growth is impaired with curvature of the weight-bearing long bones (which are not thickened). The enlarged epiphyseal plates show hollowing out or 'cupping' with an increase in depth particularly at the lateral part of the epiphysis. The diagnosis is usually confirmed on X-ray of the wrists which shows this characteristic deformity in the lower growth epiphysis of the radius and ulna. A characteristic chest deformity known as a 'ricketty rosary' occurs at the costochondral junctions as well as causing a transverse sulcus.

In osteomalacia there is rarefaction of the whole skeleton with bowing of the long weight-bearing bones. There may be multiple spontaneous crack fractures (Looser's zones) which are probably bridged by unmineralised callus. These Looser's zones provide a radiological differentiation from osteoporosis in which they are not seen. A comparison of rarefaction should be made with the hand of a normal patient, using the same exposure for both.

In all these conditions the underlying disease process should be treated, if possible, together with large doses of vitamin D, calcium and phosphorus. In coeliac disease a gluten free diet should be given and in renal tubular rickets, alkalis such as sodium citrate, are administered to combat the associated acidosis.

In addition, surgical correction of severe skeletal deformities may be necessary.

Miscellaneous conditions

Scurvy

Scurvy results from a deficiency of vitamin C (ascorbic acid). Dietary sources include fresh fruits and vegetables, with very little derived from food of animal origin. A minimum daily intake of vitamin C is 40–50 mg, and the body stores usually last for approximately 3 months, when dietary intake is inadequate.

Vitamin C deficiency produces defective collagen, which may manifest clinically as: swollen gums which bleed easily and may lead to loosening of the teeth or cutaneous bleeding in the form of perifollicular, petechial, and finally, larger bruises. There may also be bleeding from mucous membranes or into joint spaces. Subperiosteal haemorrhages in long bones may later become ossified, leading to thickening of the bones. The severe pain which results from such haemorrhages may produce a pseudoparalysis, in the acute phase. Extensive or prolonged bleeding may produce anaemia.

Characteristic radiological changes include a dense line between the metaphysis and epiphyseal cartilage, as well as ossification of subperiosteal haematomata. Treatment is with ascorbic acid supplements, followed by a balanced diet to prevent further recurrences.

Industrial poisons

A number of toxins, including arsenic, cadmium, lead, mercury, and thallium may produce heavy metal poisoning. The clinical effects of such toxins will depend on the dose, frequency, and duration of exposure. Virtually any body system may be affected. For example, lead poisoning in children may produce deposits at the growing

Miscellaneous Disorders

Scurvy

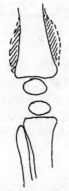

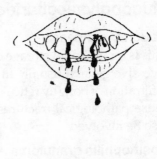

X-ray appearance of periosteal haemorrhages

Bleeding gums

Industrial Poisons

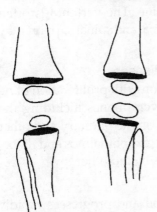

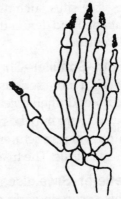

X-ray appearance of dense epiphyseal lines in lead poisoning

X-ray appearance of changes seen in polyvinyl chloride poisoning

epiphyseal plates leading to the characteristic radiological appearance of radiodense 'lead-lines'.

Certain industrial chemicals, such as polyvinyl chloride (PVC), may produce bony erosions, particularly involving the tips of the fingers and toes.

Mucopolysaccharidoses

Gaucher's disease

This is a rare lipoid storage disease due to an autosomal recessive gene. It usually first appears in adult life with infiltration of bone by reticuloendothelial cells which may cause pathological fractures. The spleen and liver may also be involved.

Eosinophilic granuloma

This is usually a solitary cystic lesion containing histiocytes and eosinophils which may cause a fracture. Surgical curettage, bone grafting and internal fixation may occasionally be required, or low dose radiotherapy to inaccessible sites such as the spine. The vertebra is often flattened and denser than normal and spinal support may be required.

Hand–Schüller–Christian disease

This is a more serious condition with proliferation of reticulo-endothelial cells in several bones including the skull. There may be pressure on the pituitary and other intracranial structures causing exophthalmos and diabetes insipidus. The treatment is by radiotherapy.

Letterer–Siwe disease

This occurs in early childhood and progresses rapidly with early death. Lipoid deposits occur not only in the bones but also in other organs including liver, spleen and lymph nodes.

Mucopolysaccharidoses

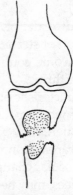

Gaucher's disease: X-ray appearance of a cystic area with pathological fracture

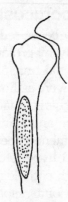

X-ray appearance of an eosinophilic granuloma

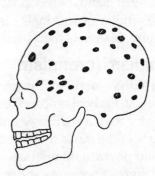

X-ray appearance of bony lesions in Hand–Schüller–Christian disease

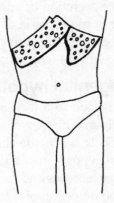

Letterer–Siwe disease

Endocrine Disorders

Cushing's syndrome (glucocorticosteroid excess)

This may be caused by an endocrine disorder or, more commonly, by prolonged administration of steroids following renal transplantation or for chronic conditions such as severe asthma or rheumatoid arthritis.

Diagnosis is usually made on the characteristic plump, florid face and pattern of obesity. In women there is usually amenorrhoea and hirsutism. There may also be associated hypertension and general rarefaction of the bones with pathological fractures. Avascular changes in the major joints, especially hips and knees, may necessitate joint replacement but these avascular changes in bones can be markedly diminished by reducing the steroid dosage.

In primary Cushing's syndrome the cause can be excessive secretion of adrenocortical hormone from a tumour or hyperplasia of the adrenal gland, or secondary to a basophil adenoma of the pituitary (Cushing's disease), either of which may require ablation of the adrenal.

Congenital hypothyroidism (cretinism)

This is due to a lack of thyroid hormone and causes dwarfism with mental retardation. Early diagnosis is essential. This is made clinically by the classic heavy dull facies, deposition of fat, the lack of the outer two-thirds of the eyebrows and mental and physical retardation.

The detection of a lack of thyroid hormone is diagnostic. There is usually dramatic improvement following the administration of thyroxine.

Endocrine Disorders

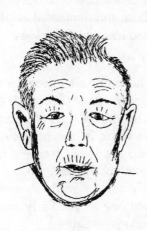

Hypopituitarism

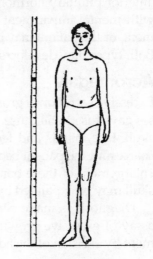

Gigantism

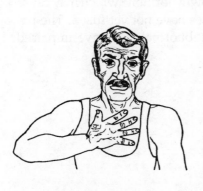

Acromegaly

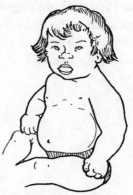

**Congenital
hypothyroidism**

Hypopituitarism

This is due to a lack of secretion of one or more of the anterior pituitary hormones. This may cause dwarfism with mental impairment and delayed sexual development, or the patient may be obese and of normal height. Both types may develop slipped femoral epiphyses .

Acromegaly

Excessive secretion of growth hormone after the epiphyses have fused will cause enlargement of the mandible, skull, face, hands and feet. The skin is thickened and coarse and the patient becomes weak. X-rays may show enlargement of these bones and the sella turcica of the skull may be expanded by growth of the adenoma.

Diagnosis is made clinically and by radio-immune assay of excessive growth hormone levels. Early treatment by excision of the adenoma is essential.

Gigantism

This is caused by an acidophilic adenoma producing excessive amounts of growth hormone which may cause gigantism if the epiphyses have not yet fused. The patient may be mentally subnormal and have impaired sexual development.

Endocrine Disorders

Glucocorticosteroid Excess

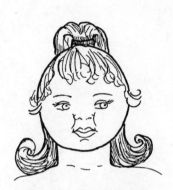

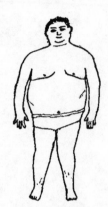

Cushing's syndrome —
'moon face' appearance

Obesity

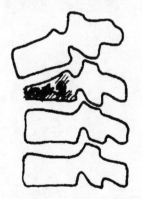

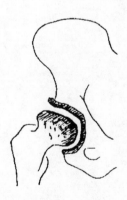

X-ray appearance of a
pathological fracture
of a lumbar vertebrae

X-ray appearance of
avascular necrosis
of the hip

A Simple Guide to Orthopaedics

Chapter 13

Upper Limb Conditions

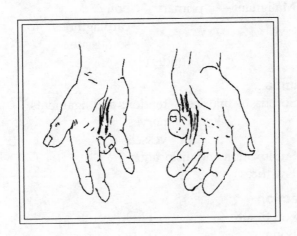

Classification

Aetiological classification

Congenital abnormalities
- Amelia and phocomelia
- Macrodactyly
- Syndactyly
- Synostoses
- Osteochondroma and other neoplasms

Neoplasia
Benign — bony
                cartilaginous
                soft tissue
Malignant — primary — bony
                          cartilaginous
                          soft tissue
                 secondary

Trauma
Soft tissue injuries — tendons and ligaments
                               nerves
                               vessels
Subluxation and dislocation
Fractures

Infection
- Soft tissue
- Bone
- Joint

Arthritis
- Degenerative (primary or secondary)
- Autoimmune

Metabolic
Haemophilic arthropathy

Paralysis

Cerebral — cerebral palsy
neoplasia
vascular conditions
trauma

Spinal — fractures
disc protrusion
syringomyelia
poliomyelitis
spina bifida

Peripheral nerves — carpal tunnel syndrome
peripheral neuritis and toxins
diabetic neuropathy

Anatomical classification

Shoulder conditions
Supraspinatus and rotator cuff
Acromioclavicular and sternoclavicular joints
Biceps tendon

Elbow conditions
Tennis elbow
Golfer's elbow
Ulnar neuritis
Olecranon bursitis

Wrist and hand conditions
Ganglion
Dupuytren's contracture
Carpal tunnel syndrome
Trigger finger
de Quervain's syndrome

Aetiological Classification

Most of the conditions affecting the upper limb are discussed in other chapters. This chapter will therefore describe only those conditions that do not 'fit' into any specific category.

The following is a summary of conditions which are described elsewhere:

Congenital abnormalities

These include deficient growth, overgrowth or fusion of limbs and various other congenital abnormalities due to genetic defects such as achondroplasia. Developmental abnormalities may also be secondary to antenatal insults such as infections, drugs and radiation.

Neoplasia

Some bony neoplasms are inherited in an autosomal dominant pattern such as multiple osteochondromata, (diaphyseal aclasis). Most neoplasms, however, are of unknown aetiology. Examples are benign neoplasms such as bone cysts and fibrous dysplasia, or malignant neoplasms such as osteogenic sarcoma, chondrosarcoma and Ewing's sarcoma.

Trauma

The differential diagnosis in many orthopaedic conditions must include old or recent injuries to bone, ligaments, tendons or other structures, which otherwise may cause difficulty in diagnosis.

Infection

Bone and joint infections may be acute or chronic and may cause osteomyelitis of bones or pyogenic arthritis of joints. Acute infections may result from organisms such

Aetiological Classification

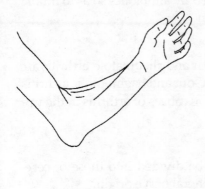

Congenital webbing of the elbow

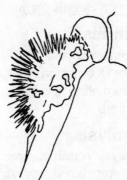

X-ray appearance of an osteogenic sarcoma

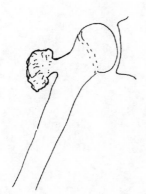

X-ray appearance of an osteochondroma of the upper humerus

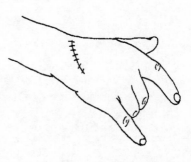

Traumatic tendon injury

as pyogenic staphylococci, whereas chronic low grade infection may be due to an organism such as Mycobacterium tuberculosis. The behaviour of an acute pyogenic organism may be modified by antibiotics so as to mimic that of a chronic organism.

Arthritis

Degenerative osteoarthritis and rheumatoid arthritis are the most common types. Gout and haemophilic arthritis are two other non-infective causes of arthritis in the upper limb.

Paralysis

Paralytic conditions can be divided into those of cerebral, spinal cord, or peripheral nerve origin.

These are described in detail in both Chapter 3 and Chapter 11.

Aetiological Classification

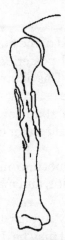

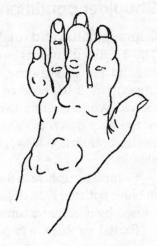

**X-ray appearance of
osteomyelitis**

Severe gouty tophi

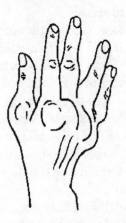

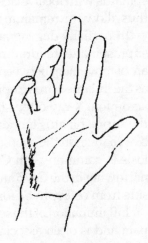

Rheumatoid arthritis

Ulnar nerve palsy

Anatomical Classification

Shoulder conditions

Supraspinatus and rotator cuff

The rotator cuff inserts into the upper end of the humerus, and particularly the tuberosity and posterior and upper part of the head of the humerus. This allows the deltoid, which inserts into the deltoid tuberosity one-third of the way down the shaft, to act as an abductor. The posterior insertion also acts as an external rotator of the shoulder.

Complete rupture of the rotator cuff is not uncommon in older patients with degenerative arthritis, and may be caused by minimal trauma.

Partial rupture also occurs, but may appear to be complete as pain limits any movement. It may be differentiated from complete rupture by injecting the supraspinatus with local anaesthetic to eliminate the pain and thus allow the remaining fibres to act.

In partially degenerated tendons, calcification in the supraspinatus tendon may occur and lead to a painful arc of movement between about 60° and 120° of abduction, as the inflamed area impinges on the undersurface of the acromion. X-ray often shows the area of calcification in the supraspinatus tendon. There may also be degenerative changes in the shoulder. Associated cervical spondylosis is common with C5 and C6 root pressure due to narrowing in the C4/5 and C5/6 foramina on the affected side from osteophytic formation.

Inflammation of the subacromial bursa may also cause pain and is often associated with degenerative changes in the tendon.

Shoulder Conditions

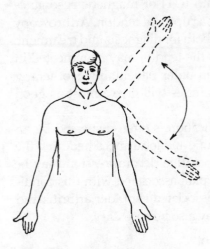

Chronic tendonitis — the
painful arc syndrome

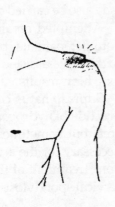

Acromioclavicular
joint subluxation

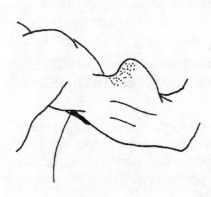

Ruptured biceps
tendon

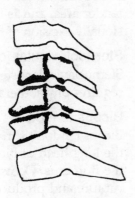

X-ray appearance of
cervical spondylosis

In addition to X-rays, and injection of a suspected partial rupture, investigations include an arthrogram, a computerised tomogram (CT) or magnetic resonance imaging (MRI) to show a ruptured tendon. Arthroscopy may also be carried out both for diagnosis and treatment.

Attempted repair of the tendon may be indicated in younger patients, but in older patients physiotherapy with active assisted exercises will give almost as good long term results.

Supraspinatus calcification is often dispersed by an injection of hydrocortisone and local anaesthetic into the area, but sometimes operative decompression may be necessary for the acute pain associated with this condition. Treatment of the associated shoulder arthritis and cervical spondylosis may also be necessary.

Acromioclavicular joint

Acromioclavicular joint osteoarthritis, subluxation or dislocation may also cause shoulder pain and limitation of abduction. It is easily diagnosed by palpation of the tender area, and is treated by physiotherapy and occasionally excision of the outer end of the clavicle.

Sternoclavicular joint

Sternoclavicular osteoarthritis or subluxation usually also requires physiotherapy and rarely operative treatment.

Biceps tendon

Biceps tendonitis may occur over the anterior aspect of the long head of biceps in the anterior upper aspect of the humerus. Occasionally a degenerated tendon may rupture and produce a painless swelling in the arm on contraction of the muscle.

Tendonitis is often relieved by an injection of hydrocortisone and perhaps physiotherapy. A rupture of the tendon is usually associated with osteoarthritis of the shoulder which is often accompanied by cervical spondylosis. The actual rupture does not cause any appreciable disability and does not require treatment.

Cervical spondylosis

This may cause referred pain into the shoulder. It is often associated with pain and numbness radiating down the arm and occasional weakness, with stiffness of the shoulder. Cervical spondylosis may also cause tenderness in the extensor muscles of the forearm. The diagnosis and treatment of cervical spondylosis is discussed elsewhere in this book (Chapter 11).

Trauma

Shoulder trauma includes fractures of the neck and tuberosity of the humerus and both anterior and posterior dislocation of the joint. This should always be considered in the differential diagnosis.

Arthritis

Arthritis of various types, including osteoarthritis, rheumatoid arthritis and gout are all discussed under the relevant sections of this book (Chapter 10).

Elbow conditions

Tennis elbow

This condition is due to a tear of a number of the fibres of the common origin of the forearm extensor muscles over the lateral epicondyle. It is usually caused by wringing of clothes and similar repetitive actions rather than tennis. There is a localised tender area, mainly over the lateral epicondyle (not the extensor muscles in the upper forearm). Gripping will usually exacerbate the pain, as will extension of the second and third fingers against resistance. Pain caused by dorsiflexion of the wrist against resistance is of limited diagnostic value.

Injection of hydrocortisone and local anæsthetic into the tender area will relieve the pain in over 80% of cases but may have to be repeated.

A support around the forearm just below the elbow is often successful. In very severe cases operation and freeing of the extensor origin is necessary.

Golfer's elbow

This occurs with tenderness over the common origin of the forearm flexor muscles and is much less common. Treatment is similar to the above.

Ulnar neuritis

This is commonly due to trauma to the nerve behind the medial epicondyle. A valgus deformity of the elbow due to a previous supracondylar fracture may also stretch the nerve. Ulnar neuritis may necessitate transposition of the nerve anterior to the epicondyle.

A Simple Guide to Orthopaedics

Elbow Conditions

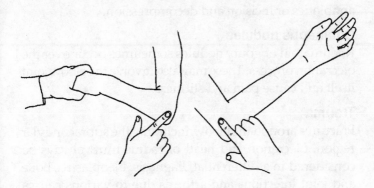

Tennis elbow

Golfer's elbow

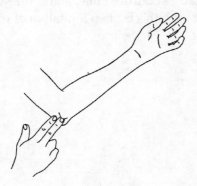

Ulnar neuritis

Olecranon bursitis (student's elbow)

This is due to pressure over the bursa which may become inflamed and infected. This occasionally requires antibiotics or incision and decompression.

Cutaneous nodules

Rheumatoid or gouty nodules sometimes occur over the olecranon process. These may also involve the elbow joint itself and cause pain and stiffness.

Trauma

Fractures around the elbow, including the supracondylar region, olecranon and head of radius must always be considered in a differential diagnosis. Neoplasms, bone and joint infections and arthritis due to various causes are discussed elsewhere in this book.

Pyogenic infection of the elbow joint itself may be secondary to an overlying wound or infected bursa, or due to systemic infection.

Osteoarthritis secondary to a previous fracture or injury often causes both deformity and stiffness of the elbow. Associated with this is often limitation of rotation of the elbow joint.

Elbow Conditions

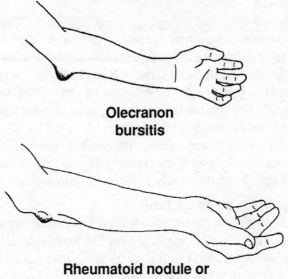

Olecranon bursitis

Rheumatoid nodule or gouty tophus

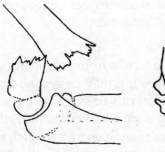

X-ray appearance of a supracondylar fracture

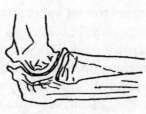

X-ray appearance of osteoarthritis of the elbow

Wrist and hand conditions

Ganglia

This is a firm cystic swelling, usually over the dorsum but sometimes palmar surface of the wrist. It probably arises from degeneration of the capsule of the wrist joint rather than a true outpouching. It is filled with glairy fluid and is firm and spherical. It may transilluminate, is only slightly tender and may disappear into the joint on extension or flexion of the wrist.

Although it may burst with trauma (the traditional cure is hitting it with the family bible!) it is best excised properly under tourniquet control if symptomatic.

Dupuytren's contracture

A Dupuytren's contracture is a fascial thickening of the palm, usually most marked over the fourth metacarpal and proximal phalanx. It may be associated with a similar condition in the sole of the foot and in the corpus cavernosum of the penis. Some drugs, especially those given for epilepsy, are sometimes responsible, as is trauma. Mild cases in the elderly may not require treatment.

In young patients, and in severe cases excision of the fibrous bands in the palm is indicated.

Carpal tunnel syndrome

Carpal tunnel syndrome results from narrowing of the carpal tunnel. This narrowing may be secondary to a previous fracture, osteoarthritis or synovial thickening in pregnancy or conditions such as rheumatoid arthritis.

The patient complains of an aching wrist, often worse at night when the arm is warm, together with variable numbness in the radial three and a half fingers and weakness and wasting of the thenar muscles.

Wrist and Hand Conditions

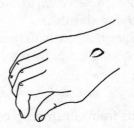

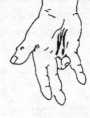

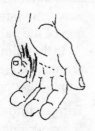

Ganglion   **Dupuytren's contracture**

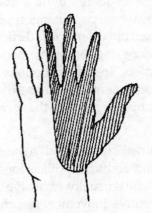

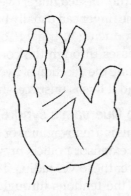

**Carpal tunnel syndrome —
thenar muscle wasting,
weakness and paraesthesia**

**Swollen hand —
tendon sheath
infection**

Rest with a simple detachable splint and anti-inflammatory drugs may give some relief but division of the flexor retinaculum of the wrist is often necessary.

Infections of the hand

Infections of the soft tissues of the hand are common. They vary from infection of the nail fold (paronychia) to infection of the palmar spaces and tendon sheaths.

In the palm, considerable swelling may occur and early drainage is essential if infection does not rapidly resolve with antibiotics.

Trigger finger

A trigger finger or thumb results from constriction of a flexor tendon sheath which produces swelling of the corresponding tendon. Repeated friction leads to localised tendon hypertrophy and nodule formation. A nodule may occasionally be congenital but is usually secondary to repetitive trauma. There is a tender nodule at the base of the affected finger over the metacarpophalangeal joint. The finger can usually be flexed but extension is difficult, producing a 'trigger' or flicking motion as the nodule passes through the constriction. Treatment options include the injection of hydrocortisone and local anaesthetic and if this is unsuccessful, simple division of the sheath.

de Quervain's syndrome

This is a tenovaginitis or constriction of the tendon sheaths of extensor pollicis brevis and abductor pollicis longus over the lower radius. The cause is usually excessive use of the tendons through repetitive movements, such as wringing of clothes.

The patient complains of tenderness over the radial styloid which is exacerbated by abducting the thumb

Wrist and Hand Conditions

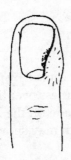

Paronychia

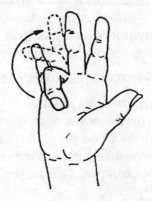

Trigger finger

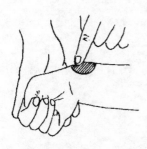

de Quervain's syndrome

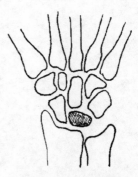

X-ray appearance of avascular necrosis of the lunate

against resistance or forcibly flexing the thumb across the palm of the hand (Finglestein's test).

The differential diagnosis includes a fracture of the radial styloid process, a fractured scaphoid or fracture or osteoarthritis of the first carpometacarpal joint.

Treatment options include injection of the area with hydrocortisone and local anæsthetic (less than 50% success) or division of the tendon sheaths.

Avascular necrosis of the lunate

(Kienbock's disease)

This is a rare condition and is probably caused by injury to the blood supply to the bone. Tenderness over the lunate will occur but the diagnosis is made on the X-ray appearance of an avascular bone which may show collapse.

Arthritis

Rheumatoid arthritis, osteoarthritis and gout are discussed in Chapter 10.

Chapter 14
Lower Limb Conditions

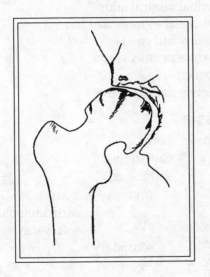

Classification

Aetiological Classification

Congenital abnormalities

Dwarfism — achondroplasia
cretinism
gargoylism
Amelia and phocomelia
CDH and protrusio acetabuli
Coxa vara and valga
Genu varum, valgum and recurvatum
Talipes
Congenital vertical talus
Talocalcaneal — navicular bar
Pes planus and cavus
Metatarsus primus varus
Macrodactyly
Syndactyly and webbing

Neoplasia

Benign — bony
cartilaginous
soft tissue
Malignant — primary — bony
cartilaginous
soft tissue
secondary

Trauma

Soft tissue injuries — tendons and ligaments
nerves
vessels
Subluxation and dislocation
Fractures

Infection

Soft tissue
Bone
Joint

Arthritis

Degenerative (primary or secondary osteoarthritis)
Autoimmune
Metabolic
Haemophilic arthropathy

Paralysis

Cerebral
cerebral palsy
neoplasia
vascular conditions
trauma
Spinal
disc protrusion
fractures
spina bifida
syringomyelia
poliomyelitis
Peripheral nerves
peripheral neuritis and toxins
diabetic neuropathy

Anatomical Classification

Hip and femur

Knee and tibia

Ankle and hindfoot

Forefoot and toes

Aetiological Classification

Most conditions of the lower limb are discussed in detail in the relevant sections of this book. It is the purpose of this chapter to discuss other conditions which do not fall into any of the other categories. Conditions discussed in other chapters are given below.

Congenital abnormalities

Developmental abnormalities include limb defects, such as overgrowth and fusion, as well as congenital dislocation of the hip and bilateral coxa and genu vara and valga.

They also include ankle and foot conditions such as talipes equino varus, congenital vertical talus, metatarsus primus varus and other foot deformities.

Generalised developmental conditions include achondroplasia and polyostotic fibrous dysplasia.

Neoplasia

Developmental tumours include multiple osteochondroma (diaphyseal aclasis) and benign bone cysts as well as multiple neurofibroma. Most tumours, however, are of unknown origin and develop in childhood or adult life. They range from benign tumours such as aneurysmal bone cysts, eosinophilic granuloma and non-ossifying fibromata, to malignant tumours such as osteogenic sarcoma, chondrosarcoma and Ewing's sarcoma.

Trauma

Various chapters discuss both recent and old injuries to bones, ligaments, tendons and other structures. It is especially important to consider trauma as an aetiological factor when dealing with swellings associated with the bone, as the differential diagnosis includes both inflammatory and neoplastic conditions.

Aetiological Classification

Congenital abnormalities

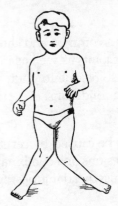

Genu valgum

Neoplasia

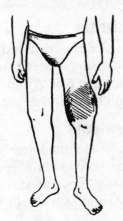

Osteogenic sarcoma

Trauma

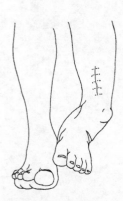

Deformity due to
tibial trauma

Infection

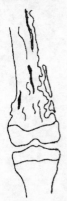

X-ray appearance
of osteomyelitis

Infection

A low grade osteomyelitis of the femur or tibia, or a pyogenic arthritis of the hip or knee sometimes is difficult to differentiate from tumours or other inflammatory conditions such as rheumatoid arthritis.

Arthritis

Osteoarthritis of the hip and knee is common and rheumatoid arthritis can occur in major joints as well as in the hands and feet. Arthritis may also be due to gout, haemophilia and other non-infective conditions.

Paralysis

Paralysis of the lower limb may be caused by cerebral, spinal cord or peripheral nerve lesions or a combination of these. They include cerebral palsy, head injuries, spina bifida and poliomyelitis.

Miscellaneous conditions

A miscellaneous group of conditions includes Paget's disease, hallux valgus and plantar fasciitis.

Aetiological Classification

Arthritis

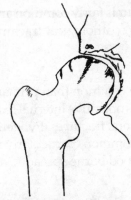

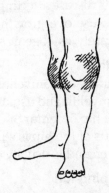

X-ray appearance of
osteoarthritis

Rheumatoid arthritis

Paralysis

Miscellaneous conditions

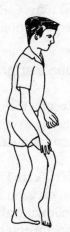

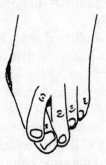

Poliomyelitis

Hallux valgus

Anatomical Classification

Hip and femoral conditions

Paget's disease
Paget's disease affecting the femur is fairly common and may cause overgrowth, bowing, pathological fractures and, rarely, osteogenic sarcoma.

Infection
Secondary osteomyelitis is more common than primary osteomyelitis and usually follows operative internal fixation of hip or femur or open femoral fractures. Pyogenic arthritis of the hip is still fairly common, particularly in children and is usually due to blood borne spread.

Snapping hip
This is a fairly common condition resulting from the ilio-tibial band catching over the greater trochanter. It may be due to unaccustomed exercise and can cause inflammation of the bursa over the greater trochanter.

This condition will usually respond to rest and anti-inflammatory drugs. It occasionally requires division of the ilio-tibial band in the mid thigh.

Tom Smith's disease and Girdlestone's arthroplasty
Tom Smith's disease is a septic arthritis of a major joint occurring in the first year of life and leading to complete destruction of the joint. It is now uncommon except in developing countries.

A similar, but more common situation, occurs following Girdlestone's procedure. This is an excision arthroplasty of the hip which is performed following an unresolved infection complicating total hip arthroplasty.

Hip and Femoral Conditions

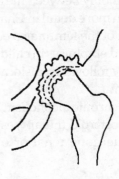

X-ray appearance of an infected hip

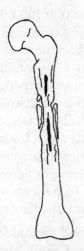

X-ray appearance of osteomyelitis

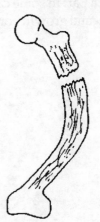

X-ray appearance of Paget's disease

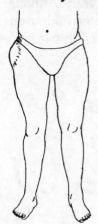

Trochanteric bursitis

Both arthroplasties may present as a telescoping unstable hip requiring later hip replacement.

Avascular hip conditions

Perthes' disease is due to avascular changes in the head of the femur. It occurs most commonly between the ages of 5 and 10 years. It is discussed in more detail in Chapter 7. Avascular changes of the head of the femur also occur in sickle cell disease and in slipped epiphyses in children. In adults, avascular changes may follow hip dislocation or subcapital fractures of the femur.

These changes also occur in chronic alcoholism and following prolonged glucocorticosteroid therapy, especially in patients who have undergone renal or other organ transplantation.

Slipped capital femoral epiphysis

Slipped epiphysis is discussed in more detail in chapter 7 and occurs most commonly between the ages of 10 and 15 years. Although trauma plays a part in some cases, in many children an imbalance of sex and growth hormones is thought to be responsible.

Hip and Femoral Conditions

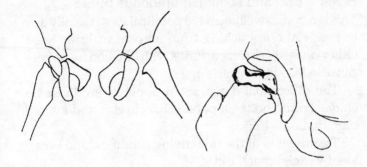

X-ray appearance of Tom Smith's disease and Girdlestone's arthroplasty

X-ray appearance of Perthes' disease

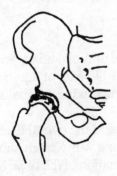

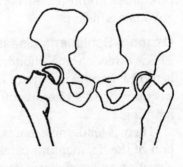

X-ray appearance of avascular necrosis

X-ray appearance of slipped capital femoral epiphysis

Knee and tibial conditions

Baker's cyst and semimembranosus bursa

This is a cystic swelling in the popliteal fossa usually due to synovial outpouching from an osteoarthritic knee. Other causes of chronic arthritis with effusion in the knee can also lead to a Baker's cyst.

The differential diagnosis of popliteal swellings includes lymph nodes, a popliteal aneurysm and a semimembranosus bursa.

Treatment is of the underlying condition and occasionally excision of the cyst.

Bursitis

Prepatellar bursitis (housemaid's knee) is due to traumatic or infective inflammation of the prepatellar bursa, that is, the bursa in front of the knee.

Infrapatellar bursitis (clergyman's knee) has similar causes.

A suprapatellar bursa is an outpouching of synovial fluid and synovia in the knee itself. It is particularly prominent in chronic osteoarthritis, and also occurs with any knee effusion.

Osgood–Schlatter's disease

This is a traction osteochondritis of the tibial tubercle and is most common in boys of about 14 years of age. Such traction injuries often result from kicking footballs or jumping.

There is tenderness and bony swelling over the insertion of the ligamentum patellae and X-ray often shows elevation and sometimes fragmentation of the tibial tubercle.

Treatment is rest from sport and sometimes a detachable splint behind the knee.

Knee and Tibial Conditions

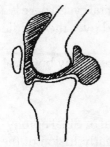

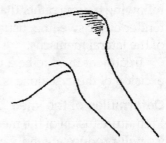

**X-ray arthrogram of
a Baker's cyst**

**Enlarged prepatellar
bursa**

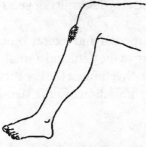

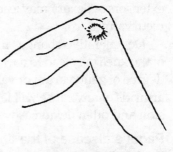

**Osgood–Schlatter's
disease**

**Lateral meniscal
cyst**

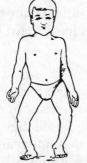

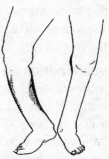

Genu varum

Paget's disease

Cyst of the lateral meniscus

This is probably a degeneration of the lateral meniscus following trauma rather than a congenital cyst. There is a tender cystic swelling, usually situated over the middle of the lateral meniscus.

Treatment used to be a total meniscectomy but local excision of the cyst alone is adequate.

Deformities of the knee

Premature fusion of the medial femoral or tibial epiphysis will produce a genu varus while early fusion of the lateral femoral or tibial epiphysis will lead to a genu valgum (Chapter 7). Unbalanced paralysis of the knee extensors or flexors may lead to flexion deformity or genu recurvatum.

Degenerative changes in the medial and lateral joint of the knee may lead to narrowing of the joint and a small degree of genu varum or valgum. Swelling of the knee in arthritis of any cause will lead to limitation of full extension and often flexion as well.

Paget's disease of the tibia

Paget's disease is discussed in further detail in Chapter 12. There is usually bowing and thickening of the tibia and pathological fractures may occur. Osteogenic sarcoma is a rare complication. High-output cardiac failure may occur in extensive Paget's disease, as the affected bone is highly vascular.

Osteochondritis dissecans

Osteochondritis dissecans usually involves the lateral side of the medial femoral condyle and occurs most commonly in adolescent boys. It usually results from trauma to the cartilage with avascular changes in the underlying bone. As a result an area of cartilage about 5–10 mm in diameter, together with the underlying bone becomes avascular. This area may detach and form a loose body in the joint, which may catch in the joint and cause it to lock.

The usual treatment is to re-attach the partially loose fragment with a recessed screw before it detaches, or excise it once it is free in the joint.

Avascular necrosis of one or both femoral condyles may occur after steroid therapy, such as in chronic asthma and renal transplantation.

Treatment is excision of the avascular segment and drilling and revascularising the remainder of the condyle. Occasionally total knee replacement is required.

Meniscal and ligamentous injuries

These may cause pain and swelling of the knee with instability and eventually osteoarthritis. Early arthroscopic excision of detached fragments or open repair is often indicated.

Ankle and hind foot conditions

Tendonitis

Tendonitis on the medial side of the ankle is usually due to inflammation of the tibialis posterior tendon sheath and on the lateral side to inflammation of the sheaths of the peroneal tendons.

Posteriorly the sheath of the tendo calcaneus may become inflamed by overuse of the tendon, by rubbing on the back of a shoe or by minor tears of the fibres of the tendon itself. Partial or complete rupture of the tendon may also occur.

Clinically there is tenderness and often swelling over the sheath of the relevant tendon and usually pain on stressing the tendon.

Treatment includes 'resting the tendon' with an elevated heel on both shoes, the application of ice packs and elevation of the leg in the acute stage.In chronic tendonitis deep heat, massage and sometimes injections of hydrocortisone and local anaesthetic into the tendon sheath (not the tendon) may be necessary. Occasionally incision of the tendon sheath may be required. Rupture of the plantaris tendon may also occur and lead to a sudden sharp pain in the mid calf. The treatment is the same as for a tendonitis of the tendo Achillis.

Painful heel

Pain under the heel is usually due to a plantar fasciitis, possibly following bruising of the heel. It may be associated with a calcaneal spur seen on X-ray but this is often unrelated to the pain. The heel sometimes becomes painful in chronic infections, in rheumatoid arthritis and in other inflammatory diseases.

Ankle and Hindfoot Conditions

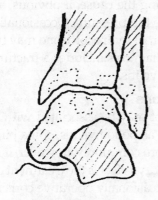

X-ray appearance of rheumatoid arthritis

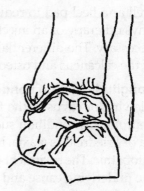

X-ray appearance of osteoarthritis

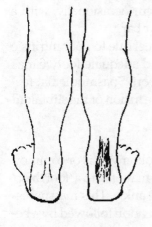

Tendonitis

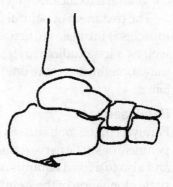

X-ray appearance of a calcaneal spur

On examination there is usually localised tenderness under the point of the heel just in *front* of the calcaneal tuberosity.

Treatment involves treating the cause, if obvious, as well as a heel pad to reduce the pressure. Occasionally physiotherapy or an injection of hydrocortisone may be necessary. The differential diagnosis includes a fracture of the calcaneus and osteomyelitis.

Longitudinal arch conditions

Clawing or cavus of the foot may be associated with a neurological condition such as poliomyelitis, spina bifida or Friedreich's ataxia. More commonly, however, it is idiopathic. The treatment of cavus feet is the treatment of the underlying cause and occasionally operative correction of the deformity.

Flattening of the longitudinal arch may be idiopathic in young patients or secondary to poor intrinsic muscles in elderly and overweight patients. Spasmodic flat feet with peroneal muscle spasm occur occasionally, with a congenital talocalcaneo-navicular bar.

The treatment of painful flat feet due to poor intrinsic muscles is intrinsic reduction and adequate footwear as well as a longitudinal arch support. Spasmodic flat feet may sometimes require operative fusion of the subtaloid joints.

Paralysed foot

Paralysis of the foot, such as in poliomyelitis or common peroneal or sciatic nerve damage, may lead to a 'foot drop' and also to a fixed equinus of the ankle. This may necessitate elongation of the Achilles tendon followed by a below knee caliper or alternatively an arthrodesis of the subtaloid joints may be needed.

Ankle and Hind Foot Conditions

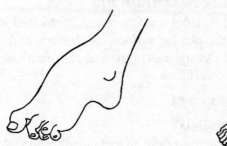

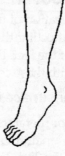

Pes cavus and clawed toes

Paralysed foot

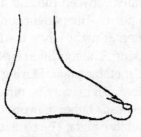

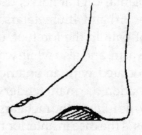

Pes planus

Arch support

Spastic paralysis from an upper motor neurone lesion may also require a below knee caliper, again sometimes preceded by elongation of the tendo Achillis.

Forefoot and toe conditions

Classification of forefoot conditions can be divided into those affecting the plantar surface, the dorsum and the sides of the feet. Deformities of the toes are often associated with these conditions.

Plantar surface of foot

Anterior metatarsalgia

This is a painful area under the metatarsal heads, commonly the 2nd, 3rd, and 4th. It is usually due to weakening of the dynamic muscular structure of the foot. It is often associated with obesity, poor muscle tone, clawing of the toes and sometimes various neurological conditions such as poliomyelitis, leading to weakness of the intrinsic muscles.

Morton's metatarsalgia (plantar neuroma)

This is due to irritation followed by enlargement of a plantar digital nerve, usually between the 2nd and 3rd or 3rd and 4th metatarsal heads. The patient complains of pain in the forefoot, often at night when the feet are warm, and also while walking. The condition is often associated with an anterior metatarsalgia. During examination the main tender area can usually be pinpointed to lie *between* the metatarsal heads rather than under them as is the case in anterior metatarsalgia. The pain is usually worse on lateral compression of the forefoot which compresses an enlarged neuroma between the metatarsal heads. There may also be numbness between the toes supplied by the relevant cutaneous nerve.

Forefoot and Toe Conditions

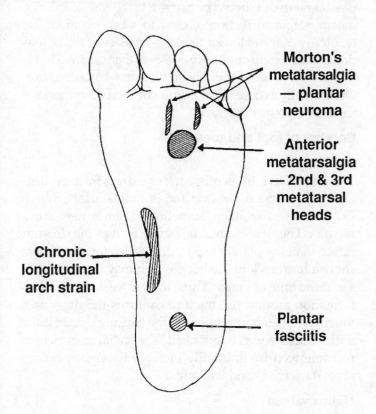

Morton's metatarsalgia — plantar neuroma

Anterior metatarsalgia — 2nd & 3rd metatarsal heads

Chronic longitudinal arch strain

Plantar fasciitis

Plantar surface of the foot

Treatment of both anterior metatarsalgia and a digital neuroma is an anterior metatarsal pad or button placed just *behind* the metatarsal heads, plus good footwear and intensive muscle reduction. If this is not successful the plantar neuroma should be excised. In the case of anterior metatarsalgia correction of claw toes by subcutaneous tenotomy of the extensor tendons, transfer of flexor tendons to the extensor or arthrodesis of the proximal interphalangeal joints of the clawed toes may be carried out. Occasionally excision of a prominent 2nd or 3rd metatarsal head may be necessary.

Dorsum of foot and toes

March fracture

This condition is often missed. It is a stress fracture, usually of the necks of the 2nd and 3rd metatarsals, due to unaccustomed walking, sometimes seen in new army recruits. The tender area, however, is over the dorsum rather than the plantar aspect of the metatarsals. X-rays show a fine crack in the bone which may be difficult to see at the time of injury. Three to four weeks later callus formation around the fracture confirms the diagnosis, much to the embarrassment of the treating doctor if the initial fracture was overlooked. The initial treatment is rest followed by gradually increased weight-bearing, graded exercises and walking.

Hallux valgus

This is a valgus deformity of the big toe which may be combined with or due to a varus deformity of the first metatarsal (metatarsus primus varus). The cause is often a combination of a genetic predisposition together with tight shoes. This causes a prominence of the first metatarsal head on the medial side of the foot which gradual-

Forefoot and Toe Conditions

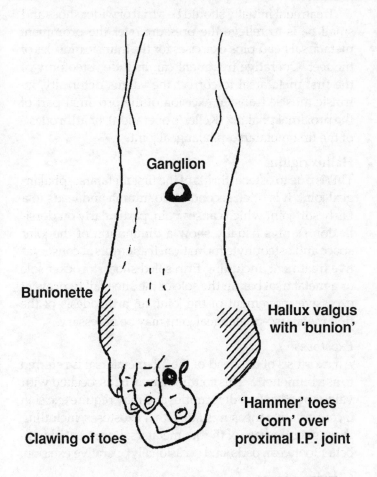

Ganglion

Bunionette

Hallux valgus
with 'bunion'

Clawing of toes

'Hammer' toes
'corn' over
proximal I.P. joint

Dorsum of the foot

ly leads to an exostosis. Overlying this prominence is a bursa which may become enlarged and inflamed to form a 'bunion'.

Treatment initially should be a trial of wider shoes and small pads to relieve the pressure over the prominent metatarsal head plus exercises for the intrinsic muscles of the feet. Operative treatment can include osteotomy of the first metatarsal to correct the valgus deformity, intrinsic muscle transfer, excision of the proximal part of the proximal phalanx (Keller's operation), or arthrodesis of the first metatarso-phalangeal joint.

Hallux rigidus

This is due to osteoarthritis of the first metatarso-phalangeal joint. It is often secondary to trauma and leads to a fairly stiff joint which causes pain, particularly on dorsiflexion. X-rays usually show a diminution of the joint space and osteophyte formation. If attempts at conservative treatment, including firm soled shoes, a rocker sole or a metatarsal bar on the sole of the shoe fail to prevent excessive movement of the joint, an arthrodesis of the first metatarso-phalangeal joint may be necessary.

Exostoses

An exostosis of the head of the 5th metatarsal is referred to as a bunionette. This condition may be associated with valgus or other foot deformities and may require excision if conservative measures fail. Other exostoses, including those over the base of the 5th metatarsal, are treated with better footwear, pads, and occasionally operative excision.

Clawing of toes

Clawing or overriding of the 2nd to 5th toes is common and is often associated with other foot deformities, or weakness of the intrinsic muscles of the feet. The 2nd toe may override a hallux valgus while the 5th toe may override the 4th. In the latter case this may be due to a symmetrical, congenital deformity. A neurological basis for clawing must always be eliminated, such as polio-myelitis, peripheral neuritis or spina bifida (especially if associated with a cavus foot and sensory deficit or motor weakness). Many cases, however, occur in elderly, overweight women with poor intrinsic muscles.

Flexed proximal and distal interphalangeal joints may cause pressure and tenderness over the end of the flexed toes which press on the shoe or ground. Correction of this condition includes appropriate footwear, intrinsic muscle reduction, 'corn' pads and occasionally operation, as discussed under anterior metatarsalgia. Other foot conditions, including exostoses, may occur elsewhere due to rubbing of shoes.

Ganglion

This is a cystic swelling filled with glairy fluid and associated with a joint. Excision of an exostosis or ganglion may be necessary if conservative measures fail and if the condition is symptomatic.

Miscellaneous conditions

The differential diagnosis of foot conditions includes congenital deformities such as talipes equino varus and spasmodic flat feet (often associated with a talocalcaneonavicular bar), tumours, trauma, infections and arthritis. All these conditions, as well as osteoarthritis, rheumatoid arthritis, gout and paralytic conditions are discussed elsewhere in this book.

A Simple Guide to Orthopaedics

Chapter 15

Orthopaedic Conditions in the Elderly

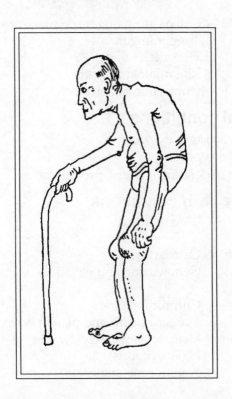

Classification

Upper limb conditions

Shoulder and arm — Rotator cuff degeneration
Frozen shoulder
Ruptured long head of biceps

Elbow — Tennis and golfer's elbow

Wrist — Carpal tunnel syndrome
de Quervain's syndrome

Hand — Osteoarthritis 1st carpo-metacarpal joint
Trigger finger
Heberden's nodes
Rheumatoid arthritis
Dupuytren's contracture

Spinal conditions

Cervical spondylosis
Senile kyphosis
Low back strain and disc protrusion

Lower limb conditions

Hip — Osteoarthritis

Knee — Osteoarthritis
Genu varum and valgum

Foot — Chronic footstrain
Plantar fasciitis and plantar neuroma
Hallux valgus and claw toes
Hallux rigidus
Anterior metatarsalgia

Introduction

It is the purpose of this chapter merely to *highlight* the *most common conditions* seen in the elderly patient and to refer the reader to the relevant section elsewhere in the book.

In the elderly, degenerative joint disease is common. Osteoarthritis may be primary due to an unknown cause or secondary to trauma, avascular necrosis or rheumatoid arthritis. Multiple repeated injuries, combined with inadequate synovial lubrication of the joints, are probably the most common aetiological factors. Total hip and knee replacements are the most common joint replacements. Where possible, the aim should be joint mobility rather than arthrodesis.

Neck and spinal conditions are often due to a combination of intervertebral disc degeneration and osteoporotic collapse.

Foot problems are commonly due to obesity and poor muscle tone. Suitable orthotic foot supports, plus physiotherapy, good hygiene and suitable shoes are all that are needed in most cases.

Degeneration of tendons may lead to rupture of the quadriceps, rotator cuff or long head of biceps. Partial tears of tendons may lead to 'tennis' or 'golfer's' elbow.

Irritation under the flexor sheath may cause conditions such as carpal tunnel compression of the median nerve and constriction of tendon sheaths leading to trigger finger or de Quervain's tenovaginitis.

Upper Limb Conditions

Shoulder and arm

Rotator cuff degeneration and frozen shoulder

Rupture of rotator cuff muscles secondary to osteoarthritis of the shoulder is common. Operative repair may be indicated in early cases of complete rupture. Frozen shoulder, often secondary to cervical spondylosis, may also occur.

Ruptured long head of biceps

Rupture of the long head of biceps may be secondary to osteoarthritis of the shoulder but causes little disability and does not require treatment.

Elbow

Tennis and golfer's elbow

'Tennis' and 'golfer's' elbow are usually due to partial rupture of a few fibres at the origins of the extensors or flexors respectively of the wrist and hand and are seldom due to sport. They can be treated by a support just below the elbow, but over 80% of patients find relief by injection of hydrocortisone acetate into the tender area.

Wrist and hand

Carpal tunnel syndrome

In elderly patients irritation of the median nerve, producing a carpal tunnel syndrome, may be secondary to a previous Colles' fracture, rheumatoid arthritis or osteoarthritis. Conservative measures such as rest may fail, and decompression of the nerve by division of the flexor retinaculum is usually very effective.

Upper Limb Conditions

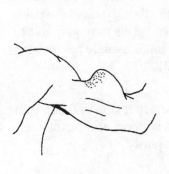

Ruptured biceps tendon

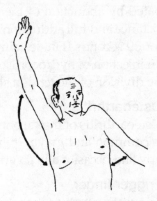

Frozen shoulder

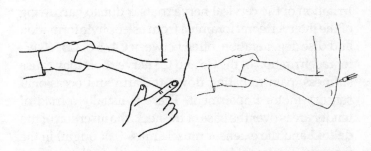

Tennis elbow

Cortisone injection

de Quervain's tenosynovitis

de Quervain's tenosynovitis is due to an inflammation or constriction of the tendons of extensor carpi radialis brevis and abductor pollicis longus over the radial styloid. There is tenderness over the radial styloid exacerbated by abduction of the wrist and thumb against resistance and full adduction of the thumb across the palm for 30 seconds (Finglestein's test). This may respond to an injection of hydrocortisone but is usually best treated by division of the tendon sheath.

Osteoarthritis

Osteoarthritis of the carpometacarpal joint of the thumb is common and may require a support and physiotherapy and occasionally an arthroplasty.

Trigger finger

Trigger finger, due to constriction of the flexor sheath over the metacarpo-phalangeal joint, may respond to a hydrocortisone injection, otherwise division of the sheath.

Spinal Conditions

Cervical spondylosis

Irritation of the cervical nerve roots is due to narrowing of the intervertebral foramina from osteophyte formation and disc degeneration, often between C4/5 or C5/6 vertebrae. Irritation of the C5 and C6 nerve roots may cause stiffness, pain radiating down the arm and occasional sensory-motor impairment. There is usually a triad of tender areas over the base of the neck, the insertion of the deltoid and the extensor muscle mass (*not* origin) in the forearm. Treatment is conservative, with analgesics and anti-inflammatory drugs as well as a collar, heat, exercises and occasionally neck traction with *rotation* and *flexion* to the affected side.

Upper Limb Conditions

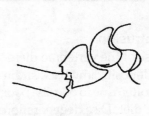

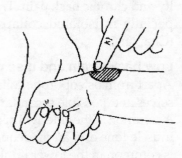

**X-ray appearance
of a Colles'
fracture**

**de Quervain's
tenosynovitis**

Spinal conditions

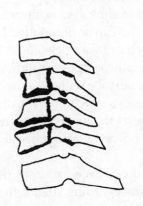

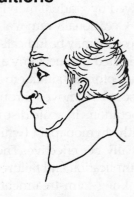

**X-ray appearance of
cervical spondylosis**

**Treatment: physiotherapy,
supportive
collar and traction**

Senile kyphosis

A senile kyphosis due to osteoporotic collapse is common, usually in the thoracic spine, and leads to deformity and chronic back pain. The differential diagnosis, especially in isolated collapse, is metastatic deposits (Chapter 11).

Low back strain and disc protrusion

Apart from osteoporotic collapse of the vertebrae themselves and possible secondary deposits, low back strain is common in the elderly. This is often due to obesity, poor muscle tone and an inadequate diet. Disc degeneration is common in the lower lumbar region, especially in the L4/5 and L5/S1 disc spaces, with irritation of the L5 and S1 nerve roots causing sciatic pain.

Treatment in the acute stage is usually conservative with bed rest, heat and exercises. Traction on both legs or the pelvis or an epidural injection of local anaesthetic and hydrocortisone for sciatic irritation may be indicated followed by gradual mobilisation with a back support.

Occasionally removal of a protruding disc causing root pressure may be indicated and this can be done either by a limited laminectomy approach or by a nucleotome. A nucleotome is similar to a knee arthroscope and allows a disc to be removed through a small tube without a major operation. In acute disc protrusions injection of the disc with chymopapain (which digests the disc) may occasionally be effective. There is, however, an appreciable complication and failure rate.

Long term treatment is by heat, back exercises (including swimming), education regarding diet, a firm mattress, upright chairs and education regarding safe lifting techniques. A back support may also be indicated (Chapter 11).

Spinal Conditions

Thoracic Spine

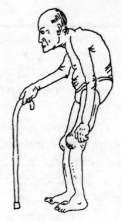

Kyphosis

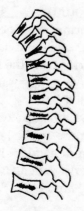

X-ray appearance of senile osteoporosis

Lumbar Spine

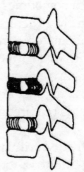

X-ray appearance of a prolapsed intervertebral disc

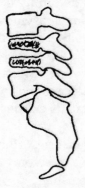

X-ray appearance of collapsed vertebrae

Lower Limb Conditions

Hip conditions

Osteoarthritis

Osteoarthritis of the hip is common in the elderly and may be unilateral or bilateral. It is often associated with osteoarthritis of the knee and low back strain due to the excessive compensatory strain caused by the flexed and adducted hip.

Physiotherapy with short wave diathermy, exercises and a raise on the heel to compensate for the flexed hip and shortened leg should be tried initially in mild cases. In elderly patients with advanced osteoarthritis a total hip replacement is the procedure of choice.

Knee conditions

Osteoarthritis and genu valgum and varum

Osteoarthritis of the knee is common, especially after a meniscus injury. This may lead to an increasing varus or valgus deformity of the knee which sometimes causes increasingly asymmetrical wear on the articular cartilages in either the medial or the lateral joint compartments. This leads to increased pain, synovitis and stiffness.

A trial of physiotherapy with short wave diathermy and exercises plus a knee support, analgesics and anti-inflammatory drugs may be all that is required in mild cases.

Severe osteoarthritis is usually treated with a valgus or varus osteotomy of the tibia or femur or a total knee replacement.

Lower Limb Conditions

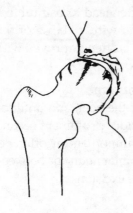

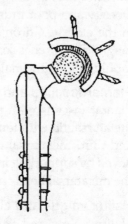

X-ray appearance of osteoarthritis

X-ray appearance of a total hip replacement

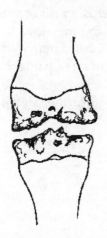

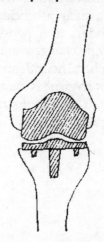

X-ray appearance of osteoarthritis

X-ray appearance of a total knee replacement

Foot

Chronic foot strain

Obesity and poor muscle tone often lead to painful feet in the elderly. Chronic foot strain with collapse of the longitudinal arch is common and is often improved with moulded longitudinal arch supports.

Plantar fasciitis and plantar neuroma

Plantar fasciitis with pain under the heel, and anterior metatarsalgia with tenderness under prominent second and third metatarsal heads is common and is often relieved by supporting insoles. A plantar neuroma between the metatarsal heads may require excision.

Hallux valgus and claw toes

Hallux valgus and clawing of the toes are often relieved by suitable shoes, physiotherapy and relieving pads, but may require operative correction.

Vascular insufficiency due to atherosclerosis or spasm secondary to hypertension or smoking may lead to ischaemic changes and ulceration. Diabetes may lead to peripheral neuritis and poor healing of sores, particularly if foot hygiene is inadequate.

Foot conditions are discussed in further detail in Chapter 14.

Lower Limb Conditions

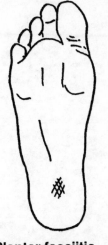

**Plantar fasciitis —
heel pad**

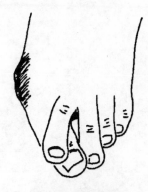

**Hallux valgus
Treatment: 'bunion' pad
or operation**

Treatment of metatarsalgia

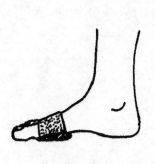

**Anterior metatarsal
support**

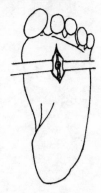

Excision of neuroma

Appendix
Reference Intervals

Haematology

Haemoglobin (Hb)	– adult male	13.0 – 18.0 g/dl
	– adult female	11.5 – 16.5 g/dl
Red cell count (RCC)	– adult male	$4.6 - 6.5 \times 10^{12}$/L
	– adult female	$3.8 - 5.8 \times 10^{12}$/L
Mean cell volume (MCV)		80 – 100 fL
White cell count (WCC)		$4.0 - 11.0 \times 10^{9}$/L

Leucocyte differential count

– neutrophils	$2.0 - 7.5 \times 10^{9}$/L
– lymphocytes	$1.5 - 4.0 \times 10^{9}$/L
– monocytes	$0.2 - 0.8 \times 10^{9}$/L
– eosinophils	$0.04 - 0.4 \times 10^{9}$/L
– basophils	$< 0.1 \times 10^{9}$/L

Platelet count	$150 - 400 \times 10^{9}$/L

Erythrocyte sedimentation rate (ESR)

–male	<50 years	1 – 7mm/hr
	>50 years	2 – 10mm/hr
–female	<50 years	3 – 9mm/hr
	>50 years	5 – 15mm/hr

Coagulation studies

Activated partial thromboplastin time	(APTT)	25 – 35 seconds
Prothrombin time	(PT)	13 – 17 seconds

International normalised ratio – INR – (therapeutic range for oral anticoagulants)   2.0 – 4.5

Fibrinogen	1.5 – 4.0 g/L
Bleeding time (in vivo test)	< 9 minutes

Clinical Chemistry

Electrolytes, urea and creatinine – (EUC's)

Sodium	135 – 145 mmol/L
Potassium (serum)	3.8 – 4.9 mmol/L
Chloride	95 – 110 mmol/L
Bicarbonate (total CO_2)	24 – 32 mmol/L
Calcium (total)	2.10 – 2.55 mmol/L
Phosphate	0.70 – 1.50 mmol/L
Magnesium	0.8 – 1.0 mmol/L
Copper	13 – 22 µmol/L
Zinc	12 – 20 µmol/L
Urea	3.0 – 8.0 mmol/L
Creatinine	0.05 – 0.12 mmol/L

Liver function tests (LFT's)

Bilirubin (total)	2 – 20 µmol/L
Alkaline phosphatase (ALP)	25 – 100 U/L
Gamma glutamyl transpeptidase (GGT) – males	< 50 U/L
– females	< 30 U/L
Aspartate transaminase – AST (SGOT)	10 – 45 U/L
Alanine transaminase – ALT (SGPT)	5 – 40 U/L
Total protein	62 – 80 g/L
Albumin	35 – 47 g/L

Arterial blood gases (ABG's)

pH	7.36 – 7.44
pO_2	74 – 108 mmHg
pCO_2	34 – 46 mmHg
Bicarbonate (HCO_3^-)	18 – 25 mmol/L
Base excess	–2 – +2
Oxygen saturation	92 – 96%

Miscellaneous

Glucose	– fasting	3.0 – 6.0 mmol/L
	– random	3.0 – 8.0 mmol/L
Total cholesterol		< 5.5 mmol/L
High density lipoprotein cholesterol (HDL)		0.9 – 2.1 mmol/L
Low density lipoprotein cholesterol (LDL)		1.2 – 4.4 mmol/L
Triglyceride		< 2.0 mmol/L
Urate – males		0.20 – 0.45 mmol/L
– females		0.15 – 0.40 mmol/L
Lactate dehydrogenase (LD)		110 – 230 U/L
Amylase		70 – 400 U/L
Acid phosphatase – total		2.3 – 5.7 U/L
– prostatic		0.4 – 1.9 U/L
Creatine kinase (CK)		
– males		60 – 300 U/L
– females		30 – 180 U/L
Alpha–1–antitrypsin		2.0 – 4.0 g/L
Iron (adult)		13 – 32 µmol/L
Total iron binding capacity		45 – 75 µmol/L
Transferrin		2.1 – 3.6 g/L
Transferrin saturation		> 20%
Ferritin	– male	30 – 300 µg/L
	– female	15 – 200 µg/L
Vitamin B12		120 – 680 pmol/L
Folate	– red cell	360 – 1400 nmol/L
	– serum	7 – 45 nmol/L

Endocrinology

Thyroid function tests (TFT's)

Thyroxine	– total (T4)	85 – 160 nmol/L
	– free (FT4)	10 – 25 pmol/L
Triiodothyronine	– total (T3)	1.5 – 2.6 nmol/L
	– free (FT3)	4.0 – 8.0 pmol/L
Thyroid stimulating hormone (TSH)		0.4 – 4.0 mU/L

Miscellaneous

Cortisol (peak diurnal)		220 – 770 nmol/L
Prolactin	– male	150 – 500 mU/L
	– female	0 – 750 mU/L

Immunology

Rheumatoid factor	
latex screen	positive/negative
nephelometry	< 50 kIU/L
Rose Waaler	< 8 U/L
C-reactive protein	< 5.0 mg/L
Serum immunoelectrophoresis	
Alpha 1 globulin	2 – 4 g/L
Alpha 2 globulin	5 – 9 g/L
Beta globulin	6 – 10 g/L
Gamma globulin	7 – 13 g/L
Immunoglobulins	
IgG	6.5 – 16.5 g/L
IgA	0.8 – 3.7 g/L
IgM	0.6 – 3.5 g/L
IgD	< 0.4 g/L
Complement	
C3	0.9 – 1.8 g/L
C4	0.16 – 0.50 g/L

References

Adams J C, Hamblen D L *Outline of Fractures*. Churchill Livingstone

Adams J C, Hamblen D L *Outline of Orthopaedics*. Churchill Livingstone

Apley A G, Solomon L *Concise System of Orthopaedics and Fractures*. Butterworths

Apley A G, Solomon L *Apley's System of Orthopaedics and Fractures*. Butterworths

Dandy D J *Essentials of Orthopaedics and Trauma*. Churchill Livingstone

Hooper G *Orthopaedics (Colour aids)*. Churchill Livingstone

Huckstep R L *A Simple Guide to Trauma*. Churchill Livingstone

McPherson J et al *Manual of Use and Interpretation of Pathology Tests* — The Royal College of Pathologists of Australasia, Sydney

Index

Note: major index entries appear in **bold** type

and illustrations in *italics*

A Simple Guide to Orthopaedics